Opening the Energy Gates
of Your Body

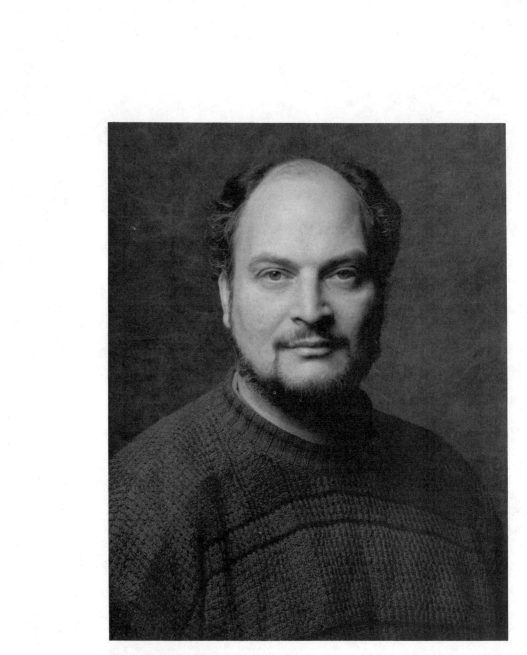

The author, Bruce Kumar Frantzis.

Opening the Energy Gates
of Your Body

Bruce Kumar Frantzis

The Tao of Energy Enhancement Series

North Atlantic Books
Berkeley, California

A Clarity Press Book

Opening the Energy Gates of Your Body

Copyright © 1993 by Bruce Kumar Frantzis. All rights reserved. No portion of this book, except for brief review, may be reproduced in any form without written permission of the publisher. For information contact North Atlantic Books, P.O. Box 12327, Berkeley, California, 94701. Printed in the United States of America.

Front cover photo by David Hiser/The Image Bank
Back cover photo by Anthony Ortega
Cover design by Paula Goldstein, Bookman Productions
Interior design by Suzanne Montazer, Bookman Productions
Illustrations by Kurt Schulten, Husky Grafx

First North Atlantic Books Printing, 1993

Published by
North Atlantic Books
P.O. Box 12327
Berkeley, California 94701

Opening the Energy Gates of Your Body is sponsored by the Society for the Study of Native Arts and Sciences, a nonprofit educational corporation whose goals are to develop an educational and crosscultural perspective linking various scientific, social, and artistic fields; to nurture a holistic view of arts, sciences, humanities, and healing; and to publish and distribute literature on the relationship of mind, body, and nature.

Library of Congress Cataloging-in-Publication Data

Frantzis, Bruce Kumar.
     Opening the energy gates of the body / Bruce Kumar Frantzis.
        p.   cm.—(The Tao of energy enhancement series ; 1)
     1. Ch'i kung. I. Title. II. Series
     RA781.8.F73   1993   92–39323
        613.7'1—dc20   CIP
     ISBN 1–55643–164–3

This book is dedicated to the wonder of the Tao, which lets all things come into being.

My profound thanks to all my teachers in the Orient, without whom it would have been impossible for me to learn and share the information presented here.

Contents

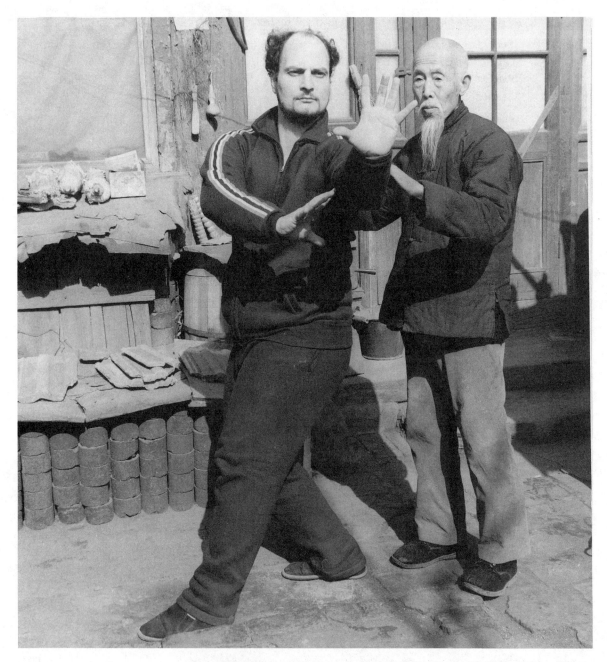

The author, training with his main teacher, Taoist Master Liu Hung Chieh, without whom this book could never have been written. The author wishes to express his deep gratitude to him for passing down the ancient traditions of Taoist meditation, internal martial arts, and Chi Gung.

Acknowledgments

My gratitude goes to many. First, to Liu Hung Chieh, a man whose intense impact on me cannot be described with words. Without Liu, I could never have learned or understood Chi Gung so completely. To all of my students, whose genuine interest was the motivation for writing this book. To Natalie Albert and Jan Lang, who first talked me into teaching them this material in the West in New York City in 1972.

Many, many people helped in the actual creation of this book. If anyone has been omitted from the following, I humbly beg their indulgence. In Santa Fe, New Mexico: David Barbero, Bernie Langan, Beverly Kune, Craig Barnes, Larry Horton, Helena Kierulf, Michael Vasquez, Donna Lubell, and Christine Richardson; in New York City: Ken Van Sickle, Susan Rabinowitz; in Boston: Bill Ryan, Eric Hoffman, and Alan Dougall; in California: Mary Christianson, Jonathan Finegold, Don Rubbo, Jim Stegenga; in Oregon, Kurt Schulten.

Special thanks go to three people: Brian Lee of Santa Fe, without whose sincere interest and prodding this volume would never have been started; Michael Winn of New York City for his support and encouragement when I was seriously considering quitting in the middle; and Stuart Kenter of San Francisco, without whom this book would never have been finished.

And for never-ending inspiration, to my wife Caroline and our wonderful boys Alex and Dominic.

Note to the Reader

The practical side of Taoism is little known in the West. Most of the books about Taoism that are available in English are broad philosophical or poetic treatises (such as those by Lao Tse and Chuang Tse) that do not reveal the actual Taoist methods by which people can manifest Taoist ideals in their daily lives.

The end purpose of all Taoist methods resides in Taoist meditation and alchemy, where an individual ultimately understands and becomes one with the mystery of the universe. Along the way, Taoists cherish practices that raise the human being from the "Inferior Man"* to the "Superior Man" of the *I Ching*, who is the only one capable of realizing the Tao.

There are many ways to refine one's body, emotions, mental and psychic energy en route to becoming—from a Taoist point of view—a mature, balanced adult. I have followed the methodology of the warrior/healer/meditator, learning along that road the martial arts, Chi Gung, Chinese medicine, and Taoist sexual practices and philosophy. Taoist friends of mine have taken the path of Chi Gung, painting, calligraphy, geomancy, and mental pursuits, including the primary method of meditation. What all Taoist practitioners of whatever Way have in common, however, is Chi Gung.

To rise from "inferior" to "superior" in the Taoist manner, the energy of one's body and emotions needs to be strong and balanced. If you are ill, Chi Gung will provide you with a means to become healthy; if your mind is disordered, Chi Gung can give you a way to attain balanced discipline and perseverance. If you are healthy, Chi Gung can raise your energy level in a

---

*The Chinese term is usually translated as "Man." Here and elsewhere in the book, we yield to this convention with the understanding that the word "Man" should be taken to mean both men and women—humankind.

balanced fashion, release suppressed talents, and prepare the body/mind/spirit to succeed in Taoist meditation. All people are born "inferior"—it is only by great effort and genuine humility that a person transcends. All sane people wish to be healthy and strong; all those interested in spirituality wish to attain their true nature. In Taoism, Chi Gung is the first basic method for achieving these very human goals.

This volume is the first of a series that contains a *complete* Taoist Chi Gung system—one that has worked for thousands of years. (Other volumes are described on page 170 in the back of the book.) This system is the foundation of the health and power abilities of both the Taoist warrior and the Chi Gung healer. By learning the practical material in this book, you will be taking the most important first step to genuine life-long health and vibrancy that it is possible to take.

If this world of ours, which at the moment is going technologically insane and spiritually bankrupt, can gain a little more internal balance from volumes such as this one, that is enough.

—Bruce Kumar Frantzis

The following material is not intended as a substitute for the advice of a physician. The reader should consult a physician before embarking on this or any health exercise program, and any physical distress during or after exercise should not be ignored, because it may indicate a health problem that requires the attention of a health care professional.

Foreword

Who Is Bruce Kumar Frantzis?

Hong Kong: In Search of the Elusive Chi Power

The dream of every serious student of Tai Chi* and Chi Gung** and the martial arts is to study with an authentic Oriental grand-master who will reveal all the secrets of these arts. These secrets of internal power are not taught to the general public, but are privately transmitted only to select family members or inner-circle disciples. In China, being accepted as the disciple of a grandmaster is the equivalent in the West of being admitted to do postdoctoral work at Harvard or Oxford with the most brilliant professor in one's field.

Bruce Kumar Frantzis is one of the very few Westerners who genuinely has been able to achieve this dream. In an odyssey through various martial arts lasting more than two decades, his ambition was always to study with a lineage grand-master. Like other Westerners who sought this path, Kumar was constantly thwarted by the tightly closed door of Mainland

*Tai Chi (pronounced tie jee) is an ancient Chinese system of movements based upon the development of the chi (life force) within the body. Cultivated chi can be used to rejuvenate the body, heal illness and injuries, maintain health, and enhance spiritual capacities. Tai Chi may also be used as a highly effective system of self defense.

**Chi Gung (pronounced chee gung) is the art and practice of internal energy development.

China, a country, throughout those years, isolated and experiencing the consequences of harsh political upheavals. His frustration was intensified by an unrelenting Oriental prejudice: the unspoken agreement that the most secret teachings should not be given to Westerners.

It was not until the summer of 1981 that one of Kumar's teachers in Hong Kong consented to give him a letter of introduction to his own master in Beijing, a man named Liu Hung Chieh (pronounced Lee'-oh Hung Jee-eh). Kumar had already been invited by the Beijing Institute of Physical Education to study Tai Chi Chuan there (*Chuan*: fist), and this letter contained potential that excited him greatly.

Beijing: The Grandmaster Liu Hung Chieh

Kumar spent mornings in the city of Beijing studying the national simplified system of Tai Chi, push hands, and weapons. The instruction emphasized the health aspects of Tai Chi over its martial arts applications, and it is here that Kumar gained a deep respect for Tai Chi as a comprehensive health care system. As we shall see, Kumar was to develop Tai Chi and Chi Gung into a viable health care program useful to the West. At the conclusion of this course, Kumar was the first Westerner to be certified by the Chinese government to teach the complete system of Tai Chi Chuan.

In the afternoons, he would go to see the 79-year-old grandmaster, Liu Hung Chieh. Liu had an intriguing past. He had lived and studied with the founder of Wu style Tai Chi, Wu Jien Chuan, and he had been the youngest member of the original Beijing Ba Gua Chang* School. When he was only in his thirties, Liu was declared enlightened by the Tien Tai School of Buddhism, after which he spent ten years studying with Taoists in the mountains of western China. He was a lineage holder in Tai

---

*Ba Gua (pronounced bah-gua) is the most sophisticated and mysterious of the Chinese internal martial arts. Based upon manifesting the energies of the *I Ching* (the Chinese *Book of Changes*), it is the only internal martial art that is one hundred percent Taoist in conception and practice. It is primarily a spiritual art that is at the same time considered to be an unsurpassed system of self-defense. It is thought by many to be the highest and the most effective of all the Chinese internal arts. (*Ba*: eight; *Gua*: trigrams; *Chang*: palm.)

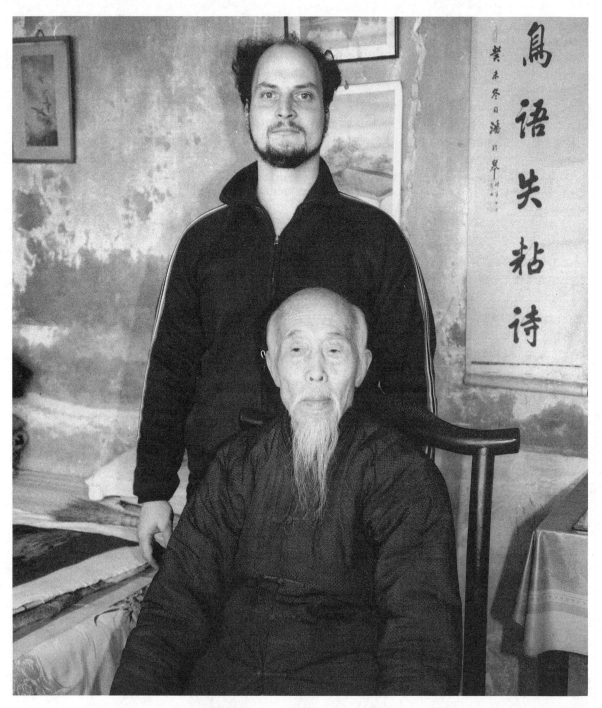

The late Taoist Lineage Master, Liu Hung Chieh, with his disciple B. K. Frantzis in Beijing, China.

Chi Chuan, Hsing I* and Ba Gua as well as an adept in Taoist Chi Gung and meditation practices.

Like many of the traditional martial artists, Liu was not a public person. In fact, since the revolution in China in 1949, he had taught Hsing I and Ba Gua to only one man—Kumar's teacher in Hong Kong, Bai Hwa. When Kumar had asked Bai Hwa if Liu would take him on as a student in Beijing, the instructor replied, "Who knows? He teaches virtually no one and it's impossible to predict what he will do."

Liu was cordial to Kumar at their first meeting. Kumar realized immediately that the twenty years he had spent immersed in the martial arts and meditation would only serve as a foundation to studying with this man. Well over twice Kumar's age and less than half his size, Liu was able to pick Kumar up and move him any way he wished. Kumar, in contrast, was literally unable to even move Liu's little finger. Kumar, considered to be a "young master" in Hong Kong and Taiwan, was duly impressed. Liu told him, "There is more to having energy than just being big."

During the years that Kumar studied with Liu, he was frequently able to observe the results of the Taoist rejuvenation techniques that the older man practiced. These would seem to change Liu from an old man to a young one in the space of a few hours or days. The transformation was amazing, and Kumar saw this control over the aging process as the mark of a true master.

Kumar requested Liu to teach him Ba Gua. Instruction entailed the severest energy work that Kumar had undertaken. After the lessons, he would be so fatigued that Liu let him lie on his own bed, entertaining him with stories of Buddhism and Taoism, and teaching him meditation. Years later, Liu revealed that the only reason he had consented to teach Kumar was that his arrival had been presaged in a dream. Liu had had five prophetic dreams in his life, all of which had come to pass. Like many of the older Taoists, Liu believed in karmic connections being fulfilled, and he felt deeply that such a connection existed between himself and Kumar. Thus, it was Liu who taught Kumar the in-

*Hsing I (pronounced shing-ee) is a major attack-oriented Chinese internal martial art based on developing chi for health, rejuvenation, and power. It is known for making practitioners physically and mentally strong, enabling them to accomplish their goals. *Hsing* means "form" and *I* means the "intention of the mind": whenever the mind moves, the body creates a form and the goal is achieved.

ternal secrets of the Chi Gung movements found in this book and the next four volumes of this series.

New York City: The First Training Ground

Born in April, 1949, in New York City, Kumar was a fat, clumsy kid who at the age of twelve witnessed a fellow student get badly injured in a fight at school. This event had a powerful effect on him, and an ad in a subway that promised "Fear No Man" led him to his first judo class. Shortly thereafter, he began to practice karate, jiu-jitsu, aikido, and Zen Buddhism.

He was fourteen when he became involved with Zen, and he used it then primarily as a means of eliminating hesitation from his karate and weapons forms. His interest in meditation at this young age was focused on using it as a tool to train the mind for martial arts rather than for spiritual growth. Even without the spiritual component, though, Kumar claims that Zen provided him with a sense of the wholeness of the mind/body/spirit and a one-pointedness that led to the strength to move through obstacles.

Consequently, his early years were concentrated on learning the Japanese martial arts. He had earned black belts in jiu-jitsu, karate, and aikido even before his first trip to the Orient, and one in judo soon thereafter. Following the recommendation of his jiu-jitsu teacher, he also studied shiatsu (Japanese acupressure massage), and he practiced this type of bodywork throughout high school. Both aikido and shiatsu utilize ki (the Japanese word for chi), or life energy; aikido for power and shiatsu for healing. So we see Kumar's interest in, and emphasis on, the subject of health started at a very early age.

By age eighteen, it had become clear to him that, in order to reach the essence of the Oriental martial, health, and meditation arts, he would have to find their source. This desire led to fifteen years of study abroad: ten years in China, three in Japan, and two in India.

By his own admission, his teenage years in the martial arts were motivated largely by a fascination with destruction. He was, at that time, preoccupied with how to injure the human body. Paradoxically, even his ongoing interest in health and meditation was, during this period, expressed in terms of violence: Zen meditation became to him a way of destroying the nonsense layers of his mind and massage a way to vanquish people's aches and pains. It was not until later, in his twenties, that he changed, allowing his interest in health and well-being to dominate completely. He became seriously involved with learning how to apply the techniques of the martial, healing, and meditation arts to preserve the useful aspects of body, mind, and spirit, keeping them from harm.

This transition began in China. Here, Kumar witnessed firsthand elderly practitioners of Chi Gung who were healthier and more vital than people half their age. He was awed, at first, by the physical power that one accrued through the practice of the physical techniques of Chi Gung. Then, when he began to learn the actual Chi Gung methods of working directly with energy, he understood: here was a way of *preserving* and *increasing* strength and vitality. He noticed that all those he saw practicing—himself included—grew stronger with age, and more content. In the hospital clinics where he worked, he watched people who had been weak and sickly all their lives become—through Chi Gung—men and women of obviously superior health and strength. He saw many who were neurotic, mentally disturbed or outright mad, or who were prone to extremes of anger, depression, anxiety or fear become calm, stable, and profound through Chi Gung. And he saw Chi Gung elevate dull minds to intelligence and perceptivity. To Kumar, the Chinese arts worked demonstrably better, and made more sense, than much of what Western medicine or athletics had to offer.

Tokyo: The Path through Aikido

In 1967, at the age of eighteen, Kumar went first to Japan, where he enrolled at Sophia University in Tokyo. His primary interest was still in the hard styles of the martial arts. He had the good fortune—from 1967 to 1969—to study with the founder of aikido, Morihei Ueshiba. Ueshiba was an extraordinary man, one who had unmistakably reached an advanced level of chi development. During the last few months of his life, too weak to walk, he was carried into the dojo (practice hall). Even in this condition, he was able to stand up and suddenly muster the energy to throw his strongest students as if they were rag dolls.

After practice, he would again be carried back to his bed. Kumar took such episodes as a graphic example of how the life force transcended mere flesh.

While Ueshiba passed on the physical techniques and spiritual philosophy of aikido to his students, Kumar felt that none of them had attained Ueshiba's superb level of chi. It had been a widely known but little discussed fact within the dojo that after Ueshiba had spent a long time in China as a monk, his entire technique changed: it went from aiki-jitsu to aikido (do is the Japanese word for Tao). That is, it went from a system based on jiu-jitsu to one based on the use of ki, or chi. At this juncture in his career, Kumar had black belts in five of the Japanese martial arts. He had visited many of the top Japanese teachers. None of them, in his view, had Ueshiba's tremendous chi power. Kumar wanted to find out what chi practices Ueshiba had learned in China.

Taiwan: The Astonishing Wang Shu-Jin*

Another experience pointed in the direction of China when Kumar visited Taiwan in 1968. There he met Wang Shu-Jin, an internal martial arts master from the city of Tianjin. Wang was in his seventies and, at five feet eight inches tall, overweight at 250-plus pounds. Nonetheless, he proved to be physically quicker than the much younger Kumar, whom he could throw or knock across the room at will.

In their first conversation, Wang maintained that karate had inferior fighting technique and insisted that actual prolonged karate practice itself would make your body old and damaged before its time. Kumar, who had studied karate for most of his life, disagreed vehemently, which resulted (as such differences of opinion between martial artists often do) in a challenge. Wang invited Kumar to test the reality of his view.

Kumar recalls that he only ended up hurting his hands and feet on various parts of Wang's body, and he especially remembers Wang's disconcerting habit of ending up behind him several times during the fight, tapping him on the shoulder. Etched deeply in Kumar's mind is the moment in their match when

---

*Wang's name is written as Wang Shu-Chin in many English language publications.

Wang walked slowly toward him, eyes half shut. Kumar relates that he actually began to fear for his life. He backed up against a wall, braced himself, and heel-kicked Wang as forcefully as he could in the solar plexus. The kick simply woke Wang up and made him mad. He tapped Kumar on the head. Kumar felt a bolt of electricity jolt through his body and the next thing he knew, he was suddenly, and to his complete surprise, on the floor.

Kumar began to practice with Wang's five A.M. class in Tai Chung Park. About a week into the sessions, a fellow student, an old man, asked Kumar if he wanted to "play." The elderly man was short and thin, a student after all, and Kumar felt a bit uneasy, not wanting to take advantage of the man. He acquiesced, however, and after being hit a few times, decided his concern was misplaced. He went after the old man as hard as he knew how. The fellow had no trouble handling Kumar as an opponent. Kumar was stunned at this turn of events. While he was standing there dazed, the man's wife came over and asked if *she* could have a go. After a year in Japan, Kumar did not know how to refuse such offers. He found to his amazement that she could spar with him on the level of any top competitive Japanese second-degree black belt in karate.

Kumar became so utterly depressed over this experience with the elderly couple that he seriously considered quitting the martial arts completely. That Master Wang Shu-Jin could beat him was one thing; that these seemingly average students could beat him was something else again. He had been a black belt for four years by this time. He had been training in Japan for eight hours a day. Yet he felt he had missed the boat. Were they going to bring out five-year-olds to beat him next? Should he have started when he was three instead of twelve? Should he have been practicing *fourteen* hours a day?

He had the opportunity, a few days later, to converse with this elderly couple from Taiwan. (By then Kumar was fluent in Japanese, which many elderly Taiwanese spoke.) They showed him some before-and-after photographs. They had come to study with Wang seven years previously because the man suffered greatly from arthritis. He was initially concerned with regaining his health, not with learning martial arts. After three years of practicing Tai Chi, Ba Gua, Hsing I, and Chi Gung, however, he was loose and straight and felt he could cease practicing. Six months after he stopped, his symptoms recurred. When he resumed practice, the symptoms went into remission.

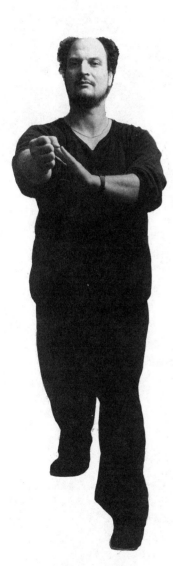

Kumar executing an internal martial arts punch.

The day before this conversation, trying to regain some of his lost confidence, Kumar had fought—and was duly beaten by—some of Wang's teenage students. It became more than obvious to him that *all* of Wang's students had reached a superlative level of both health and power through chi development. Kumar's thought changed direction: if each and every one of Wang's students could attain these ends, then he could too. His commitment to study the Chinese internal arts with Wang was cemented then and there.

Wang began to explain the difference between the internal and external martial arts. Whereas the external arts develops the bones, muscles, and outer physique, the internal arts concentrates on the development of chi. Chi Gung and the internal arts of Tai Chi, Hsing I, and Ba Gua enable one to work with the energies of the body, so that chi becomes as tangible as a solid object. The energy field in the air becomes as real to a Chi Gung or internal art practitioner as the water in the ocean is to a swimmer.

Before the internal arts were ever used for self defense, they were part of Taoist yoga, where their chief purpose was to heal the body, calm the mind, promote longevity, and form the physical foundation for higher meditation practices. The internal arts are based on beautiful flowing movements that develop structural integrity, sound body mechanics, and a strong sense of physical and psychic power. The nineteen-year-old Kumar would never forget the words directed to him by the seventy-year-old Wang: "I can eat more than you can, I have more sexual vitality than you do, I can move and fight better than you can, I never get sick, and you call yourself healthy? There is more to being healthy than merely being young. Chi can teach you all of this." Kumar recognized the truth in Wang's words and studied with him on and off for ten years.

Kumar returned to Sophia University in Tokyo. From 1968 to 1971, while still taking courses there, he pursued his study of the internal arts with the Hsing I master Kenichi Sawaii and with various students that Wang Shu-Jin had in Japan. He was also fortunate enough during this period to have encountered an old Chinese doctor who taught him Chi Gung Tui Na (pronounced chee gung twei na), a Chinese bodywork system whose fundamentals he was able to learn within two years. (Kumar was to learn much more about this system over time and to use it in his clinical work.) With this doctor, Kumar had for the first time found a man who could consistently transmit the chi energy from his own hands to cure illnesses and repair the bodies of others. During his third year in Japan, Kumar became a special karate research student in Okinawa, where he concentrated further on karate and weapons systems. Here, at the veritable birthplace of karate, he keenly felt the absence of practices that developed chi and improved health, as well as a lack of many of the most sophisticated martial arts techniques. He came to a realization that caused him to give up study of the purely external hard styles for good. From this point on, he focused all his efforts solely on the internal martial arts and Chi Gung.

India: Meditation as Chi Cultivation

From the Taoism that he had learned from Wang Shu-Jin in Taiwan, Kumar knew that energy cultivation can be one of the basic methods of meditation. Since legend dictated that Bodhidharma had brought the martial arts and meditation from India to the Shaolin Temple in China in the fifth century A.D., Kumar, always an avid seeker of original sources, decided to go straight to the Indian source. (He had been unaware of the historical fact that China possessed both martial arts and a highly honed chi development methodology centuries before Bodhidharma's visit.)

In 1971, after four-and-a-half years in the Orient, he came back to the United States. Deeply disappointed by the Oriental teachers he encountered in America (as he saw it, they either withheld information, or did not have genuine knowledge to impart in the first place, or were unable to convey what they did have because of language difficulties), he decided to return once more to Asia, the "Harvard" of energy development. Until 1987, when he anchored himself permanently in the United States, Kumar spent the years alternating between Asia and the West. He earned his living by teaching Chi Gung and the internal martial arts in the United States and Europe and practicing the healing art of Tui Na as well. In 1972, after a six-month stint of teaching Tai Chi to Americans, he departed for India.

He went first to an ashram in southern India to learn the techniques of pranayama yoga,* which works directly with the life energy. He practiced in the classical manner—using breath,

---

*Prana: breath; *yama*: to control or develop. Pranayama is the Indian parallel to Chi Gung. Beginning with breath control techniques, one eventually learns in this practice to control the internal life force energy movements through concentrated thought.

mantras,† and mudras‡—four sessions a day, three hours a session. After three months of this intensity, Kumar says that he was "able to awaken the Kundalini shakti," a spiritual force that purifies the consciousness, eventually resulting in enlightenment. In northern India, he studied Tantric Kundalini meditation with Guru Shiv Om-Tirth of Rishikesh, an experience that enabled him to comprehend the fundamental energetic similarities and differences between the Chinese and Indian systems of energy development.

Kumar knew that both the Indian and Chinese practices, if implemented correctly, could heal disease and increase longevity through development and control of the life force. Both systems had been proven by the test of time and both had undergone literally thousands of years of testing and refinement. The main difference that Kumar perceived between the two systems at the level of health resided in the nature of their practice: the Chinese system is concerned with body motion, the unceasing flow of energy, like water in a stream, whereas the Indian methods use postures with distinct beginnings and ends, and pauses between each posture. This difference is more profound, on an experiential level, than it might seem. Tai Chi is active; yoga is passive. Yoga seems to give greater flexibility, whereas Tai Chi builds greater power and integration of movement. Yet both are similar in that genuine Hatha yoga teaches pranayama with the postures—the postures open the body and the pranayama works with the energy. Genuine Chinese internal arts, in comparison, utilize certain movements—motions that encourage internal energy circulation. But without internal energy work, the amount of energy gained in either system is relatively small. Kumar believes that, in the vast majority of instances, the teaching of yoga and Chi Gung in the West fails to include the internal components. Sole emphasis on the external martial arts, or the external movements of Tai Chi, or the external postures of yoga, Kumar maintains, can only develop a severely limited amount of chi.

The two systems are by no means mutually exclusive. Kumar believes that they can be practiced simultaneously to beneficial effect. For those who are currently practicing yoga, the

---

†Chants using specialized sounds that cause specific energies to be released at the physical, mental, and spiritual levels.
‡Hand and finger positions that evoke energies and mental states in the practitioner.

Chinese arts can prove a wonderful adjunct, accelerating the process of clearing obstructions and developing energy. Kumar, however, though eventually able to achieve many of the most difficult postures of Hatha yoga, never found this practice as satisfying as the movement arts.

There was one aspect of his India experience that Kumar felt uneasy about: the concept of the Guru. Worship of the Guru plays a pivotal role in the Indian traditions, the Guru being God's direct representative on earth. As divine agents, gurus are treated with a deference and reverence that very few Westerners would accord to a living person. Though the Chinese tradition also accords a greater respect to teachers than one finds in the West, Taoist masters (bear in mind that not all Chinese masters are Taoist) are considered to be more or less custodians of ancient wisdom. The relationship between student and teacher in the Taoist way is more like a respected friend helping a friend than a godlike master helping out a mere mortal. The Taoists consider everybody to be one in the Tao and they speak of being friends in the Tao. Consequently, Kumar's training under the Taoists had a much lighter feeling for him than his training under the gurus.

In India, then, Kumar was able to formulate a comparative perspective on the world's two classic systems of internal energy. He assimilated a great deal of valuable knowledge on meditation and chi there. He also picked up a nearly fatal case of hepatitis.

Taiwan, Hong Kong, Poona, Beijing: From Consummate Fighter to Consummate Healer

The extremely virulent form of hepatitis Kumar contracted in India killed two close friends and left his own liver severely damaged. He is convinced that without the energy work learned from Tai Chi and Chi Gung he too would have died in India. His situation was grim. He lay on a hospital bed barely able to move. The Indian doctor who examined Kumar told him that he was in danger of dying. He recognized the truth of what the physician said and knew that he would in fact die unless he did something. He crawled out of his bed and, shaking all the while, he stood and forced himself to do Tai Chi and Chi Gung movements. The pain throughout his body was fierce, but he persevered until he finally collapsed back onto the bed. He slept continuously for three days. When he awoke, he knew that he would live.

When he was able to travel he returned to Taiwan. Here he practiced the internal arts with a passion, working with Ba Gua fighting master Hung I Hsiang for four years over time. Kumar is certain that this practice slowly regenerated his liver, allowing him to continue his martial studies. He explored the half-internal, half-external Kung Fu styles of the Eight Drunken Immortals, Northern Praying Mantis, Fukien White Crane, Northern Monkey, and Wing Chun. He realized that many of the truly superior martial arts teachers from mainland China were very old, and felt that this might be his last chance to learn many of these arts well, before they faded completely from the face of the Earth.

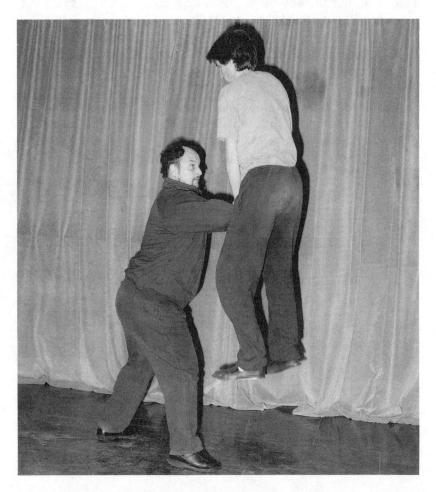

Kumar discharges energy in order to uproot his opponent. This is an advanced technique commonly found in Tai Chi Chuan Push Hands practice and other internal martial arts.

During this incredibly intense period of concentration on the fighting arts, Kumar squeezed out time to study medical Chi Gung for treating specific diseases. He paid special attention to Chi Gung for nerve and spine regeneration. With his energy level continually increasing from his practices, he was also able to devote time to studying meditation with Taoists, whose emphasis was on clearing negative emotions from the body and the mind.

Toward the end of 1975, Kumar flew back to Manhattan, teaching semi-privately and treating a small group of patients with Chi Gung exercises and with Tui Na. He was still unwilling to teach publicly, both out of respect for the Oriental tradition and because he felt that fundamentally he did not know enough to teach in this way—he would not be able to monitor the progress of his students over time, as he wanted.

In the United States this time around, he became acutely aware of the significance of stress in American life, and of the vast numbers who were burning themselves out through overwork and worry. He thought a great deal about how to apply his Taoist learning to this problem but knew that there were gaps in his medical education. Many of the internal organ and structural health problems he encountered were beyond his abilities to deal with as a Chi Gung healer. He kept a careful log of all the weak areas in his training and when he returned to the Orient within a year, he attempted to find the missing medical links he required.

His search for insight into the emotions and their impact on stress-related conditions took him to Poona, India, in 1977. There, he continued his Tantric studies while simultaneously working with a group that explored the connection between emotions, the psychological realms, meditation and chi, integrating Kundalini methods with New Age psychotherapeutic techniques. This research provided Kumar with excellent information on how the workings of the Western mind fit into the Oriental energy framework.

He was back in Taiwan in late 1977, devoting twelve hours a day to the internal arts, refining what Ba Gua he knew, immersing himself in Taoist and Tantric meditation, and developing a sharp interest in processing bound emotional energy. He continued his work with the spine and nervous system, completing an advanced acupuncture degree in Hong Kong in 1978 but choosing to concentrate on Chi Gung therapy instead of further practicing acupuncture.

In late 1979, he moved to Denver, Colorado, opening a private school that was restricted to a few continuing students. (It was not until after studying with Grandmaster Liu in Beijing that Kumar was confident enough of his mastery of the internal components of Chi Gung to teach public workshops and author books on the subject.) After enjoying considerable success in the full-contact fighting arena for years, Kumar now began to shift away from fighting to focus with more depth on healing and meditation. Though at the end of the 1970s and through his subsequent years in Beijing Kumar continued to refine his fighting techniques, his emphasis had markedly and irrevocably changed. In Beijing, in the summer of 1981, the seminal time when he worked diligently with Grandmaster Liu Hung Chieh, he was so entrenched in his training he never even visited the Forbidden City, even though it was a five minute walk from Liu's house.

In fall of 1981, Bruce Kumar Frantzis returned to Denver, where he quietly resumed teaching—to train instructors—and was nearly crippled for life.

Denver: The Crisis of Self-Healing

In early 1982, Kumar was involved in a bad automobile accident. He suffered massive injury to his spine. Two vertebrae were badly cracked, a few more had hairline fractures, many of the spinal ligaments and tendons were torn, and all his vertebrae were knocked out of alignment. Surgeons pressured him to have a spinal fusion which Kumar, through his pain, impolitely refused. His years of exposure to Chi Gung and Tui Na had taught him that, given his condition, once his spine was cut open, the chi of his body would never be as full again. Keeping the surgeons at bay, Kumar began doing Chi Gung flat on his back eight to ten hours a day.

Miracles did not occur. It was a long, hard ordeal regenerating his spine with these techniques. Complications arose. Kumar speaks of how the shattering of his spine neutralized every psychological control mechanism he had. All the darkest forces suppressed in the depths of his mind surfaced. Without his years of centering work in meditation, Kumar was sure that he would have gone over the edge, sentenced to life in a mental hospital. Instead, he held on.

But the emotional experience on top of the constant nerve pain made life unbearable, for himself and for those around him. His sudden loss of physical strength and ability, the broken pride as an athlete, was a devastating blow. He fell into an abysmal depression, losing all interest in Tai Chi and unable to do Ba Gua because of the pain. He knew he had to do something about his mental outlook. The feeling of being useless to himself and his students could not continue. When the Chi Gung finally repaired his spine so that he could move to some extent, Kumar participated in various mind/body therapies in Colorado and Oregon. They helped somewhat, reinforcing his mental stability. However, no matter how effective a psychological therapy may be, round-the-clock nerve pain creates emotional havoc. The psychological work was not enough.

Kumar tried all the physical therapies, including chiropractic, deep tissue work, Rolfing, acupuncture, massage, and a variety of movement therapies. They, too, helped marginally, abating the pain for a day or two. But it always returned. When it became clear that the alternatives available to him in the West would not permanently restore him, Kumar did what he had always done—he went to China to search, this time for the appropriate healing technology to make his own body whole.

Beijing Again: The Final Lesson with Liu

Summer, 1983. Liu was in meditation retreat and unavailable when Kumar arrived in Beijing. Another letter from Bai Hwa, his teacher in Hong Kong, enabled Kumar to study the inner technology of Yang style Tai Chi with Lin Du Ying* in Xiamen, Fujien Province. Though Kumar had studied the Yang style of Tai Chi with many teachers, including Yang Shao Jung (the greatgrandson of the original Yang, who founded the Yang style of Tai Chi) he had great respect for Lin Du Ying, deeming him the most exceptional practitioner of the Yang style he had ever seen. Since Kumar had been accepted as a formal disciple, he was given the information openly. He felt that it was an honor to be allowed to receive the Tai Chi transmission from Lin.

*Lin Du Ying was a disciple of Wu Hui Chuan and Tien Jau Ling, both of whom were top students of Yang Pan Hou, son of Yang (Lu Chan), who originated the Yang style of Tai Chi. Lin Du Ying taught the Yang style in a very pure manner, in much the same way as it was taught a hundred years ago, before it became diluted.

八卦掌师傅系统表.

一代 董海川

二代 尹福 馬維祺 程廷華

三代 馬貴 李永慶 劉標庄

　饅頭郭 程有龍

四代 朱文豹

五代 劉振麟

六代 劉洪俊

七代 白樺 范親仁

KUMAR FRANTZIS

其餘本門師友尚多不及
备載，僅擇其尤要而又有
：直接系统者錄馬
1981.9.9.

The Ba Gua Chang certificate of lineage held by Kumar.

When after nine months Liu was finally free, Kumar joined him. While his practice of the Yang form had eased the pain in his neck and upper back, the rest of Kumar's body still hurt. Liu prescribed Wu Style Tai Chi. This style emphasizes soft healing and meditation; it strengthens the body and clears the mind. Within months, practicing the Wu form obliterated the pain in Kumar's middle and lower back.

Liu then began teaching Kumar Taoist meditation, twice a day, in two to three hour sessions. Once Kumar's lower back had healed sufficiently, Liu commenced the teaching of Ba Gua and Hsing-I, as well as certain Chi Gung methodologies. This training went on for three years, seven days a week, nonstop.

Liu filled in many gaps in Kumar's esoteric education (accumulated over twenty years) and escorted him to places in the mind he never knew existed. He led Kumar through all the levels of Taoist meditation practice, directly to experiencing the place where all is unified with the Tao. It was Liu's wish that Kumar teach not only martial arts and Chi Gung (which, by this time, he was thoroughly qualified to do), but Taoist meditation as well, when Kumar felt comfortable to do so. It was through Liu that Kumar was able to organize the Chi Gung system presented in this remarkable series of volumes. Liu took the unprecedented step of authorizing a Westerner to impart knowledge locked up in China since antiquity.

On December 1, 1986, Liu died one day after he finished teaching Kumar the last palm change of Ba Gua Chang and the final level of Wu style Tai Chi. He had passed the lineage on to Kumar. The sadness, for Kumar, was overwhelming. He felt deeply privileged to have met such a man. To have studied with Liu was to have been the recipient of a great and rare gift. After being extended the honor of stirring Liu's ashes, usually an act confined to the immediate family,* Kumar returned home to the United States.

Kumar's goal in the West is to convey as much as possible of the life-enhancing material he has learned. Liu's generosity gave Kumar knowledge and confidence, and it is Kumar's hope that he can bridge cultures by making this knowledge available to people in the West. "The time for secrets," Kumar says, "is past."

Stuart Kenter, Series Editor

*Liu had officially adopted Kumar as his son in a Confucian ceremony.

Introduction

Chi and Chi Gung

What Is Chi?

Put simply, it is that which gives life. In terms of the body, chi is that which differentiates a corpse from a live human being. To use a Biblical reference, it is that which God breathed into the dust to produce Adam. Chi is the basis of acupuncture; it is the life energy people try desperately to hold onto when they think they are dying.

A strong life force makes a human being totally alive, alert, and "present," while a weak life force results in sluggishness and fatigue. Energy *can* be increased in a human being. Consequently, the development of chi can make an ill person robust or a weak person vibrant; it can also enhance mental capacity.

The concept of "life force" is found in most of the ancient cultures of the world. In India, it is called prana; in China, chi; in Japan, ki; in Native America, the Great Spirit. For all these cultures, and others as well, the idea of life force is or was central to their forms of medicine and healing.

What Is Chi Gung?

Chi Gung, which literally means "energy work," is the practice of learning to control the movement of the life force internally, using only the mind to direct energy in the body. Physical movement may be used, but is not required. The Chi Gung practices presented in this series of volumes include many of the ancient

Chinese techniques for increasing life energy. Increased life energy, in turn, manifests in a variety of ways, from improved physical health to greater mental clarity and spiritual attainment. In fact, regular practice of these exercises will lead to a body/mind that is functionally younger, so that one's "golden years" are truly golden, rather than rusty.

China's 3000-Year-Old System of Self-Healing

The effectiveness of Chi Gung has been proven in China by its beneficial impact on the health of millions of people over thousands of years. Developing the life force, or chi, is the focus of Taoism, China's original religion/philosophy. The Taoists are the same people who brought acupuncture, Chinese herbal medicine, bone setting, and the yin/yang concept to the world. Unfortunately, most of the specifics of these valuable contributions have until just recently been blocked from Western awareness by immense cultural and language barriers. These barriers are beginning to break down to an extent in acupuncture, but with regard to Chi Gung they are still very much in place. This series of five volumes on the methodology of Chi Gung is devised to help knock down these walls.

For most people, the first and foremost benefit of Chi Gung lies in the relief or prevention of chronic health problems. The range of maladies that have been helped by Chi Gung in China include cancer, internal organ problems, poor circulation, nerve pain, bad backs, joint troubles, and general physical disease.

Chi Gung Gives Mental Clarity

Of course, many physical problems are at least partially due to, or aggravated by, mental/emotional stress, so the importance of the inner tranquility developed through Chi Gung cannot be overestimated. The practice of Chi Gung helps manage the stress, anger, depression, morbid thoughts, and general confusion that prey on the mind when its chi is not regulated and balanced. Strengthening and balancing the energy of your mind enhances your ability to detect subtle nuances and to perceive the world and its patterns at ever-increasing levels of complexity. People who do not practice some form of energy development may never acquire these abilities.

The Three Spritual Treasures of Chi Gung

Chi Gung is also useful on the spiritual level. The ultimate aim of all inner Taoist practices is alchemical transformation of the body, mind, and spirit, leading to union with the Tao. Feeling the energy of your body makes it possible for you to understand the energy of your thoughts and emotions, and this leads to comprehending the energy of the spirit. From here it is possible to fully understand the energy of meditation or emptiness, and through emptiness it is possible to become one with the Tao.

According to Taoism, every human being contains "the three treasures"—*jing* (sperm/ovary energy, or the essence of the physical body), *chi* (energy, including the thoughts and emotions), and *shen* (spirit or spiritual power). Wu (emptiness) gives birth to and integrates the three treasures.

The Taoists use the all-pervasive life energy as the basis of spiritual investigation. The ultimate goal, becoming one with the Tao, has been called many things, such as "enlightenment," "meeting with the Father in Heaven," "reaching Nirvana," and "ultimate understanding." The Taoists feel that it is best for one to begin with the energy of the body, then progress through emotions and thoughts to spiritual power, before going for the ultimate.

Popular opinion has it that once you have reached a state of emptiness, you stay there, but this idea is false. You merely become increasingly familiar with this state, and learn how to spend more and more time there. As long as you live in a physical body, physical needs continue to exert demands, and dwelling completely in emptiness is not possible. Taoism has developed advanced techniques to work with the energy of wu.

Chi Gung can be practiced by individuals who only want to become physically healthy, and could not care less about psychological or spiritual matters. For generations, Chi Gung has been used by martial artists, many of whom remained unconcerned with spiritual development. Nonetheless, all Taoist spiritual practice begins with Chi Gung practice, no matter what level of attainment one wishes to finally achieve.

Energy Blocks Can Be Cleared with Chi Gung

Many people involved with spiritual disciplines focus their attention on enlightenment, and in the process injure their bodies and agitate their minds. They attempt to train in the higher spiritual disciplines without first clearing the energy blocks in their physical and emotional bodies. This way of proceeding can cause the equivalent of a short circuit in their systems, as spiritual practices generate more power than their bodies or minds can handle. Many monks from different Buddhist sects in China have had to seek out Taoist masters to repair the damage to their systems caused by overly forceful meditation techniques.

Many practitioners of spiritual methods progress with agonizing slowness *because* their physical or emotional bodies are blocked. Ironically, it is this forced slow pace that saves them from getting burned out or physically hurt. The practice of Chi Gung, or similar energy techniques, can remove these energy blocks and accelerate spiritual progress in a safe and sane way.

Chi Gung Is a Complete System of Personal Development

Chi Gung represents a *total* system of energy work. The exercises presented in this first volume are all that are necessary to maintain high-level health and increase overall awareness. This set of exercises can also serve as warm-up exercises for the internal martial arts. These will give the average person as much internal benefit as they would likely obtain from the practice of Tai Chi with the vast majority of the Tai Chi teachers in the West, as most teachers either do not know or do not share information regarding the internal workings of Tai Chi. The five volumes of this series contain, in an extremely concentrated form, all of the most important and health-giving components of Tai Chi's energy system.

Chi Gung Builds Athletic and Martial Arts Power

Chi Gung is the basis of the power of the Chinese martial arts, whether Kung Fu, or the more subtle internal forms, such as Tai Chi, Hsing I, and Ba Gua. It is almost impossible to determine from an external view how the seemingly gentle, smooth movements of the internal forms enable the advanced practitioner to defeat the most violent street fighter. This capability is basically derived from the practice of Chi Gung, which develops chi and internal power.

People who train in the internal martial arts will find that practicing the material revealed in these five Chi Gung volumes will enable them to pass far beyond external movements or athletic ability alone.

Chi Gung Is Not an Athletic or Religious Cult

The United States and Western Europe are presently besieged by cults. Generally speaking, people involved in Chi Gung do their best to avoid cultish identification. Chi Gung is something you do, something that benefits your life. It is not you, you are not it.

For five thousand years, Taoists have practiced techniques for developing chi. Most modern Taoists are reluctant to publicly declare that they do so. The phenomenon of cults is something China has seen many times and has deemed to be nonessential in terms of human evolution and the development of consciousness. Use Chi Gung to make your body more healthy, your mind more clear and balanced, your emotions more calm, and to increase your spiritual capacities. Do not make the practice of Chi Gung yet another wedge that divides people into groups of those who do and those who do not.

The Mind Directs the Chi

The science of Chi Gung is based on the axiom that the mind has the ability to direct chi, and in these volumes you will learn how to accomplish this. You will learn to feel your central nervous system, which is the intermediary between thoughts and chi. Anyone practicing Chi Gung can begin to feel their nerves, and this ability increases with time. You will literally learn to go inside your body with your mind, feel what is there, and direct your chi where it needs to go. This is not a mysterious process, but a natural one that can, with time and effort, be acquired.

It is possible to get 50 to 60 percent of the potential health benefits of Tai Chi just by doing these exercises, which are probably only one-tenth as difficult to learn as Tai Chi. Above and beyond the health benefits of Chi Gung, there are higher level techniques in Tai Chi, which are accessible only after mastering all the internal material of these Chi Gung exercises.

Relationship of Chi Gung to Tai Chi

In the West, most systems of Tai Chi or other internal martial arts are taught from the viewpoint of movement, with principles such as softness, relaxation, and body alignment thrown in. However, most of the internal components of Tai Chi that bring about health, are commonly (even usually) overlooked. Whether this lack of information is due to the reticence of teachers or the language and cultural barriers between China and the West, the point is that a large vacuum of knowledge does exist for Westerners. This series of five volumes fills that vacuum. The fundamental information available herein is far from common knowledge.

The traditional and complete internal martial arts of Tai Chi, Hsing I, and Ba Gua are extremely subtle and advanced forms of Chi Gung. Again, authentic material on these arts is rarely found in the Western world and, where it is found, the transmissions tend to be clouded.

There Are Many Benefits to Group Practice of Chi Gung

As Tai Chi is often performed in groups, so, too, Chi Gung can be done by the young and the old together, to the mutual benefit of both. In Western society at present, young, middle-aged, and elderly people do not spend very much time with each other on a person-to-person basis, without hierarchical constraints. Lack of respect among differing generations, with the old generally considered worthless and youth worshipped, is one of the results of the baby boom "me" generation in the United States and Europe. If different age groups avoid spending leisure time together, the tendency toward separation (an "us" and "them" mentality) will naturally grow.

In China, it is quite common to see a group of about 200 people practicing together, about half over 60 and other ages evenly represented. When people practice Chi Gung, they tap into their inner nature, and after practice it is very common to see the different age groups engaged in friendly conversations, usually related to Chi Gung. Because everyone has been exchanging energy on a subtle level, the barriers between people are easily dissolved, which has kept a generational harmony among Chi Gung groups in China that is virtually unparalleled anywhere else in the world.

The value of Chi Gung, both individually and societally, has been proven by millions of people in China, in one of the most crowded environments the world has ever known. As such, it could easily meet the needs of the West, with its overcrowded cities and incredible stresses.

These Chi Gung Exercises Are Safe for All Ages

When these exercises are done on their own, they are among the most time-efficient and powerful exercises anyone, regardless of age, sex, or physical aptitude, is likely to find. They can rejuvenate the elderly. (Actually, more than 50 percent of the people who begin Tai Chi and Chi Gung in China do so after the age of 60, when the realities of aging can no longer be pushed aside.) Hundreds of millions of people over the age of 60 have found Chi Gung to be uniquely effective. If a form of exercise can make the old functionally younger, its effect on the young or middle-aged is inestimable. If nothing else, it is guaranteed to help release stress, as well as improve your sex life.

These particular Chi Gung exercises can even be adapted for use by the bedridden in hospitals. They are quite safe. Anyone can do them. Such is not the case with many other types of Chi Gung, which without the constant supervision of a teacher may have a significant damage rate.

The chi flow in the body may be likened to an electrical system. If there isn't enough insulation on the wires, or the circuits are connected improperly, the system can short-circuit or otherwise malfunction. You do not want this happening to your body.

There are hundreds of Chi Gung systems, but the techniques they use (which have countless names) can be boiled down to five or six basic types. Some Chi Gung systems require that a teacher meet regularly with no more than a few students at a time in order to preclude potential damage. There are Chi Gung systems that must only be begun before puberty. There are methods that are inappropriate for certain groups to practice, such as males, or females, or people with specific health problems, or people of certain emotional dispositions, or people who have been injured physically or mentally. The exercises presented in this series are the best that could ethically be put in print for the general public. These exercises can be practiced without trouble by almost anyone, which is as safe as any Chi Gung system gets.

The Coming Medical Crisis in the West

Until about 1980, the medical systems of the United States and Europe ran reasonably well. Traditionally, the over-60 population fluctuated at somewhere below 10 percent of the total population. Older people require significantly more medical attention for the same illness than younger people do—people in their 30s with liver problems, possibly even caused by alcohol, might need a week or two in a hospital, but a person over 60 could need four to six weeks for the same problem. The deterioration of our medical system is partly due to this simple fact.

As the population of elderly has consistently risen in the United States, the American medical system has approached a state of collapse. With each percentage point rise, hospital administrators wonder when the system is going to fail completely. When approximately 15 to 18 percent of the population passes the age of 60, the problem will most likely have reached crisis proportions.

The result of such a situation is "medical rationing," which will be even worse for the elderly.

According to the National Institute of Aging (NIA), new ways must be found to enhance and maintain fitness among the "old-old" (beyond age 75) because recent statistics paint an alarming picture of their physical condition: 40 percent cannot walk two blocks; 32 percent cannot climb ten steps; 22 percent cannot lift ten pounds; 7 percent cannot walk across a small room; 50 percent of older people who fracture hips never walk independently again and many die from complications.*

Health Insurance Does Not Guarantee Good Health

Insurance companies keep increasing their rates dramatically, for as the percentage of people over 65 rises, the number of claims also rises. Within fifteen years or so, people who are not part of the corporate structure may not be able to afford to buy insurance unless they are inordinately wealthy.

One health insurance carrier favors the idea that all second opinions must go through *their* company doctors, meaning that *their* doctors would have the final say in deciding whether some-

*From Linda B. Downs, "Tai Chi," *Modern Maturity* magazine, the official publication of the American Association of Retired People, June–July 1992.

one gets potentially expensive help. It is not hard to see where a conflict of interest might arise in this situation. When a large percentage of the population is over 60, you may well need a doctor to be a relative or a friend in order to be examined. Consider the cultural revolution in China, during which the intense shortage of medical personnel meant that doctors could quite easily have an official caseload of 400 patients a day. Under these conditions, some pretty grim stories emerged. In seeing a doctor, politics and connections counted for a lot more than the severity of the illness. The fact was that many with a genuine need could not be tended to by people in the medical professions.

This discussion leads to some very basic questions, which any Westerner should seriously consider. For example, is my health my responsibility, or the responsibility of others? Can I trust my health to insurance companies, who potentially have an excellent financial reason to make my medical care less than it could be? Will I be denied health insurance, period? How will I feel when I have to enter an old-age home? Do I genuinely want to be physically and mentally active in my later years, and am I willing to put in the time and effort—through Chi Gung—to achieve this? Is it worth daily practice? Can I deal with something like Chi Gung long term, without being hung up on instant gratification?

The Chi Gung Solution to China's Medical Crisis

After the revolution, China found itself with less than half of its former medical personnel, both Western and traditional. The rest had been killed, fled the country, or gone underground. During the Mao era, the population increased from 400 to 800 million.

The government acknowledged the crisis. Having no interest whatsoever in facing a counter-revolution, leaders took draconian measures. Fortunately, what they implemented worked. The national health problem stabilized until the needed quantity of medical personnel was finally attained.

What the government did was this: they told the top Tai Chi teachers that they must design Tai Chi and Chi Gung programs for the health of the general population. Many of these masters wanted to keep their secrets to themselves, so their families could retain their "patents." It has been said that the government insisted that they make their secrets public, or face the extermination of their families down to the last child or relative. Given traditional Chinese family values, this would have loosened things up significantly, and a national program of Tai Chi, incorporating many of the principles in these Chi Gung volumes, was set up across the country.

Nonemergency patients visiting hospitals with complaints from chronic illnesses caused by poor lifestyle or overwork were directed to the hospital administrator. There, they were provided with an ID card and given the name of a nearby Tai Chi or Chi Gung practitioner. If patients wanted to qualify for another doctor's appointment, or admittance to a hospital, they were required to have their card stamped every day for three months by the Tai Chi or Chi Gung instructor, certifying they had practiced. It must be remembered that the only access to medical care was through the government—there were few, if any, private doctors in China at this time.

The system worked. Tai Chi and Chi Gung managed to keep health matters as stable as they could be kept given the poor sanitation and starvation diet most lived with. For the Chinese to get through this incredibly rough period, from the mid 1950s on, it is estimated that between 100 and 200 million people practiced Tai Chi or Chi Gung daily. (Chi Gung is currently becoming more popular than Tai Chi in urban environments, because space keeps getting tighter in China, and Chi Gung requires less room.)

Tai Chi and Chi Gung are the only internal energy systems that have actually worked for large masses of a population. Yoga practitioners never really exceeded one percent of India's population. The ancient Greek mystery schools never extended to more than one-tenth of one percent of the Greek population. Considering the parallels between the problems presented by the West's aging population and what China went through, there is much encouragement that Chi Gung methods can serve as one way to prevent a great deal of the medical misery that our increased elderly population will most certainly be confronting. This is not merely opinion: the demographics are there—the medical crisis in America will eventually manifest. Socialized medicine alone is not the answer; many European countries with socialized medicine are facing the same problems. Aging populations that require high-tech medical care simply create too much expense to bear.

The Benefits of Chi Gung vs. Western-Style Exercise

Most exercise in the West, such as jogging, swimming, bicycling, and so forth, works primarily on the muscles (including the heart) and the lungs. The Chinese also partake in Western-style exercise, but Chi Gung is thought to be of a higher level. Why? The following sections answer this question explicitly.

Chi Gung Loosens the Muscles and Builds Power

Chi Gung works with the muscles quite differently than typical exercises do. Aerobics and vigorous stretching build strength and flexibility; Chi Gung and other internal exercises build effortless power and looseness. The feeling of strength, of being "pumped up," obtained in Western exercise is actually due to muscular contraction, and even though you may be able to do leg splits, for example, this kind of contraction prevents the free flow of chi.

In the internal arts, the feeling of strength is considered inappropriate; the goal, rather, is a feeling of relaxed power. Relaxed power comes when the muscles, rather than fighting and straining to do something, just loosen (open up) and allow the energy to flow through.

Chi Gung Strengthens the Organs

The Chi Gung techniques discussed in this series—especially the Swings—work to strengthen and balance *all* the internal organs. There are also other techniques (not mentioned in this book) to strengthen *specific* organs: to help the liver recover from hepatitis, for instance, or the lungs from tuberculosis, or the heart from a heart attack. Even without having had a serious illness, almost everyone is born with a weakness in one organ or another, and Chi Gung has exact exercises to address an individual's problems.

Chi Gung Improves Cardio-Pulmonary Function

Most people think that aerobic exercise is necessary to strengthen the heart and lungs. While aerobic exercise does accomplish this, so does Chi Gung. Slow, deep, regular breathing and energy movement combine to work oxygen deeper into the tissues than regular exercise.

One case in point: One Chi Gung student who holds a normal, sedentary office job and engages in almost no aerobic activity has a brother who is a well-known mountaineer. Invited to climb a mountain in Colorado with his brother, he imagined himself gasping for air as his brother marched ahead, but much to his surprise he found that his capacity for physical activity, in terms of breath, had actually come to surpass that of his brother, who engaged in aerobic activity continuously.

Chi Gung Strengthens the Nerves

Chi flows primarily along the nerves of the body. Although at advanced levels of development chi and the nerves can be felt separately, the great majority of beginners only have awareness of their nerves.

The nerves are an intermediary between the body and the mind, and it is through the nerves that we are used to gaining information about our body. Much of the initial Chi Gung work, which emphasizes getting in touch with the body and clearing out blockages, is accomplished through the nervous system. As your chi gets stronger through continued practice, your nerves are strengthened and your body awareness is enhanced. People with poor coordination and other motor problems can benefit greatly, and everyone is aware of the important role spinal nerves play in overall health. The entire chiropractic system is based on the importance of spinal nerve flow.

Chi is also an intermediary between the body and the mind, and while it travels with nerve impulses, it can, with practice, be felt independently. It is commonly said in the internal arts that the mind moves the chi, and the chi moves the body. This is true, but it is important to be aware that most beginners need to work through the nerves first.

Chi Gung's ability to strengthen the nervous system makes it a magnificently effective technique for relieving stress on a day-to-day basis, as well as rebuilding bodies that have broken down due to long-term stress.

Chi Gung Improves Vascular Function

Western aerobics increase circulation by exercising the heart. Chi Gung improves circulation by increasing the elasticity of the blood vessels themselves. It is standard in China to prescribe Chi Gung exercises for both high and low blood pressure, as both are due to problems in vascular elasticity and strength.

Chi Gung Can Be Used by the Seriously Ill

Western exercise utilizes either motion or resistance to motion to strengthen the body (for example, weight lifting, calisthenics, running). Unfortunately, the seriously ill and bedridden often do not have the capacity for vigorous exercise. This means that the muscles and organ systems get weaker during prolonged bed rest, and it may take months to get back to normal after recovery from the main problem (a back injury, say). Chi Gung, however, has many techniques specifically designed for the weak and immobile, techniques which increase physical capacities without requiring movement.

In China, Chi Gung is also prescribed for terminal cancer patients as a last resort. If they don't initially have the strength to practice while standing or sitting, they practice lying down until their strength builds up.

Chi Gung Eases Stress and Balances Emotions

Much of the new literature on stress indicates that one of the largest factors in determining stress level is the emotions. Most physical exercise is at least somewhat useful for relieving anger, but one need only look at the behavior of some top athletes to see that typical physical activity is not the answer.

The clearing process in Chi Gung can be used on strongly repressed, as well as on spontaneously expressed emotions. Many of the movements of Chi Gung can be refined to specifically address your problem area, be it depression, grief, frustration, irritability, or any combination thereof.

Stress-related problems in our society are worsening, so it is urgent to gain the ability to convert such energies to those that are positive in nature. The ability to release stress directly through control of the central nervous system is a method *par excellence* for dealing with "burnout."

You Can Teach Chi Gung to Your Friends

Once you know this material, by all means teach what you are sure of to your friends. Of course, you don't want to start teaching it to others until you've gained a certain level of competence and inner knowledge.

The elements of standing meditation are quite safe, assuming you abide by the 70 percent rule (see page 83). Demonstrate the standing meditation to anyone who is interested. (The movement exercises are more problematical, and you should really have your movements checked by a qualified instructor before you teach them to others.)

Be guided by the old maxim: do unto others as you would have them do unto you. Be clear with anyone you teach regarding the extent of your knowledge, and don't teach what you don't understand. You may have managed to avoid pitfalls, but until you are quite familiar with the subject, you may not be able to help others do the same.

With this in mind, we welcome you now to the extraordinary world of Chi Gung.

How Chi Gung Works

The Internal Mechanics: Chi Gung and Body Health

The Blood Is Circulated without Stress on the Heart

Chi Gung works strongly on the body fluids, including blood, lymph, and the synovial and cerebro-spinal fluids. Concerning the circulation of blood, the object of Chi Gung is not to make the heart pump more strongly, but to increase the elasticity of the vascular system. As the vessels expand and contract with more vigor, the heart doesn't need to pump as strongly, which provides it with more rest. Thus, the beneficial consequences of Chi Gung, and the internal martial arts, are primarily vascular, rather than cardiac, in nature.

The Lymph Pump, Hence the Immune System, Is Strengthened

The lymph fluids are moved primarily by tiny muscular contractions. The Chi Gung techniques taught here employ some of their strongest motions where the largest lymph nodes are located; that is, the armpits, the backs of the knees, and the inguinal region. The relatively fine muscular contractions improved by Chi Gung move lymph efficiently through the entire system. These actions, as well as the overall increase in chi that Chi Gung brings, *strengthen the body's immune response.*

The Synovial Fluid Is Vitalized, Bringing Flexibility to Joints

Synovial fluid is found in the joints. It lubricates the joints, allows joint flexibility, and when functioning normally helps prevent arthritis and rheumatism. From the point of view of Chinese medicine, when "wind/damp" or physical obstructions (coagulated blood, calcium deposits, and so on) get stuck in the joints, the results are not only specific joint problems but a decrease in the flow of chi through the entire body as well. Chi Gung works with the synovial fluid by compressing and expanding it, preventing and reversing all sorts of joint problems.

The Cerebro-Spinal Pump Becomes Efficient

Cerebro-spinal fluid is basically a nutrient bath and lubricating liquid that surrounds the spinal cord and brain. It keeps a constant pressure in the human body. This pressure regulates nerve flow and affects every physical sense. All the Chi Gung techniques in this series of volumes help strengthen the cerebro-spinal fluid pumps in the body and add chi to the cerebro-spinal fluid itself.

The quality of your physical senses is determined by the health of your spine. Your cerebro-spinal fluid, to a great degree, determines just how healthy your spinal cord is, and how efficiently the spinal nerves carry messages from your brain to your body and from your body to your brain. All Chi Gung work strongly affects the cerebro-spinal pump, both by physically pumping the fluid and by moving chi, all of which encourages the cerebro-spinal fluid pump to perform at optimal efficiency.

The Muscle Tissue Gains Elasticity

Chi Gung also causes muscle tissue to elongate. This activity differs from stretching in the usual sense. The object here is to fill the tissues with energy, so that they stabilize at a given degree of stretch. With most forms of stretching, the body soon shrinks back to its original state when the stretch stops. With the stretches of Chi Gung, however, the muscles eventually attain a state akin to that of a springy rubber band. A few athletes possess this muscular springiness naturally, but anyone can attain this state with Chi Gung practice.

The Tendons Are Strengthened

Chi Gung also adds greater strength and elasticity to the tendons. This contributes to the tremendous flexibility many Chi Gung practitioners have, which derives primarily from the tendons and ligaments, not from the muscles. Chi Gung has the ability to not only make ligaments more springy but also to shrink and stabilize overstretched ligaments, which make a joint too floppy—a problem experienced by many dancers.

The Bone Marrow Is Energized

Chi Gung affects the bones by directly infusing the bone marrow with energy. This technique is an advanced one, but by the time a disciplined practitioner reaches an advanced level of Chi Gung, the energizing of the bone marrow has started to occur.

Body Cells Are Healed

Masters of Chi Gung have been healing people suffering from chronic or incurable diseases since ancient times. In modern-day China, there are sections of hospitals and clinics that use Chi Gung to treat conditions unresponsive to other methods of therapy, such as acupuncture, Western medicine, and herbs. Here patients learn to regulate their own chi, with a little help from their therapist. The range of maladies amenable to such treatment is quite broad, ranging from nerve diseases, such as Parkinson's, to cellular diseases, such as cancer.

The Process of Awakening Chi in Your Body

Your Body Will Awaken in Stages

If you constantly practice Chi Gung, your body will open up in layers. Muscles that were initially numb will begin to regain sensation. Your body will begin to reveal itself to you gradually, in a marvelous process of discovery. As your body becomes more alive, you'll be able to feel how your physical self works from the inside out.

It is not farfetched to say that you may actually begin to feel your internal organs (kinesthetically sense where your liver and spleen are, say) and what they are doing at any given time (as opposed to knowing this information intellectually). This sensitivity allows for detecting potential problems well before they ever get to the point of causing trouble.

The Body-Awakening Process Is Irregular

The process of opening the body is more often like an uneven roller coaster than a linear journey. One week one part of your body will open; the next week another part will open, while a previously open part closes again. The process is a bit like a game of "now you see it, now you don't." The time will come, though, when your body will open up and stay open, completely accessible to your awareness.

Never Force Open Body Parts That Are Blocked

What happens if you encounter, and cannot get rid of, a particular block during the standing or some other exercise? The answer is simple: Do not force it. Rather than remaining at that one unmovable block and working away at it fruitlessly for a prolonged time, just move on to the next step. You may find that the next day or week the immovable block will quite suddenly dissolve.

Your Chi Is Growing Even if You Cannot Feel It!

What happens if you practice Chi Gung for a while but don't feel anything different going on in your body? This is in fact the case for many people. It takes time for you to become sensitive to the chi, but a good rule of thumb to go by is as follows: If you find yourself feeling more comfortable, or if you are able to do more things without strain, or if you do not get sick as much as you used to, or if you start developing a type of effortless concentration and ability to do physical things you never before even thought were possible—your chi is growing whether you are aware of it or not. Keep practicing and you will eventually feel the chi in a very real way.

Strange Sensations Are Normal

Some of the common sensations people report when they feel the chi starting to move in their bodies include: feelings of warmth, extreme heat, electricity, heaviness, lightness, expansion, contraction, pressure, an internal sense of wind or water moving.

Chi Gung Frees Trapped Emotions

When energy enters your system it affects every level of your being. Some of its physical effects have already been mentioned. However, as the chi grows stronger in the body, it also charges up emotional energies.

Large numbers of people in the West are extremely repressed emotionally, as they have spent a great deal of time and effort learning to control emotion. Emotions that have never been expressed stay in the energy body of a human being at the fringes of conscious awareness. As you open up the chi flow in your system, the chi can give emotional energy more power, just as it strengthens your physical energy.

Increased emotional energy enables you to feel your present emotions, as well as those you have suppressed for a long period of time. Emotions such as anger, fear, love, hate, sadness, or joy may arise for no apparent reason. Often during practice, or more commonly a few hours after, such feelings, severe in nature, may suddenly appear. It is important to understand that these sensations, which we call emotions, do not require acting out—just experience them internally and let them wash through you.

If a person feels angry and takes it out on someone else either physically or mentally, the anger may actually increase rather than be expended. However, if the dissolving techniques taught in Chi Gung are used on the emotional "body," that same anger can then be transformed into a healthy, usable form. Behaviorally acting out negative emotional energy that was stuck to begin with may further entrench it. Again, understand that nothing has to be "done" with this energy. You can merely monitor it as it dissolves and is reassimilated and turned into a healthy constructive force. On the energetic level, it is just as unhealthy to throw emotional energy around externally as it is to repress it.

Taoist and Western Psychotherapy Compared

Kundalini and Group Therapy Approaches

The Taoist view of the transformation of emotional energy differs radically from the cathartic practices of either Eastern Kundalini or Western group therapy. In the kundalini practice, catharsis is sometimes called *kriya*, or action. Here, the idea, in the early developmental stages, is to discharge emotional energy by various actions, such as screaming, yelling, crying, curling into the fetal position—moving through blocked emotional states until they are freed up. In group therapy (from primal scream to encounter, bioenergetics, and psychodrama) the idea is to emote your pain and agony externally, the louder the better, heaping verbal and physical abuse on a pillow or a person, as the case may be. Though these approaches are sometimes successful, the Taoists had previously detected an inherent problem with them.

When pressure builds up in a pressure cooker, there are—within the cathartic model—only three options you have to handle the situation: (1) turn the heat off (i.e., deny, repress); (2) let some steam out at intervals; or (3) let all the steam out at once. Turning the heat off leaves the basic emotional situation unchanged. The trouble with letting steam out partially is that, after a period, the pressure will build to again reach a critical level. All the "steam" can be let out of a trapped emotion at one blow, but the reality is that this particular event rarely occurs. Far more common for people with emotional blockages is that they let some, but not all, of the emotional pressure out, and then—as mentioned—the pressure rebuilds until they have to "cathart" again.

The cathartic release of violent emotions irritates and exhausts the system, and can also foster an addictive need to feel violent emotions in ever-stronger forms. Cathartic methods may easily turn their practitioners into therapy junkies—angry people become angrier still, for instance, or depressed people sink deeper into depression, while throughout they delude themselves into thinking that they are having a good time working on improving themselves.

Taoist Therapy Emphasizes Dissolving Emotions into the Chi Flow

The Taoists found that emotional energy can be manipulated more or less like physical energy. Thus, Taoist practices are based on allowing emotional energy to move through your system until it completes itself; there is no attempt to push the energy out or to prevent it from occurring in the first place. The principles are quite similar to what one finds in acupuncture. In acupuncture, when a needle is first inserted into a point in the body, the needle may vibrate as it encounters blocked energy. When this blocked energy finally breaks through and continues moving on its path, the needle then stops shaking. It does not matter how powerful the energy going through the line (or meridian) is; what is important is whether or not it gets stopped or blocked.

Therefore, simply let the emotional energy that comes up find its way through your system. If the emotions are too strong for you to handle, follow the same pattern suggested for dealing with a block in the physical body: namely, back off and try to dissolve the block again later, so that it diminishes slowly over time. Attempting to resolve the situation in one great extremist heroic effort will not work, and will cause a lot of unnecessary misery.

Emotions are only sensations, which we then designate as good or bad. The sensations themselves are fairly neutral. Chi Gung practitioners learn to differentiate between frequencies of energy that are intrinsically benevolent to their emotions (but nonetheless can evoke thoughts, even uncomfortable ones, that have to be dealt with) and energy running through the emotional body that is essentially malevolent; that is, out and out destructive to the overall energy system.

What to Do if Emotional Difficulties Persist

If the practice of Chi Gung opens too many emotional doors at once, causing difficulties,* you can, for example:

*Such as hallucinations, emotional disturbances, or nervous breakdowns. These situations rarely occur in practice and are most prone to manifesting in people who have a history of psychological or emotional problems.

1. Contact a genuine Chi Gung or meditation adept who can instruct you on how to run energy through your system in a way that will be productive to you. Such teachers may also provide you with subsidiary practices that will benefit your specific situation.
2. Talk to somebody you trust and love, and see if they can help.
3. Try contacting some sort of psychological therapist, who may be able to help you. However, if this is a genuine body energy problem, purely psychological methods may not be enough.
4. Contact a religious counselor or psychological support group and see what help they can give.
5. Please refer to Appendix C for more information.

The arising of emotional issues during the practice of Chi Gung is a positive sign. It is far better to move through old emotional blocks than to go through life emotionally shut down. It is significantly healthier to learn to dissolve, on a daily basis, the negative emotions you are constantly exposed to than absorb them and then abuse your spouse, child, dog or anyone else who happens to be around you.

It is my hope that the emotional-release function of Chi Gung, almost unknown in the West, becomes common knowledge. It is extraordinarily powerful, humane, and gentle, and could prove of great value in the Western World. Chi Gung for emotional energy transformation is not dramatic, just effective.

Cultivate Your Chi Slowly and Safely

All safe chi development practices are cumulative and progress slowly, developing strong links between the brain and the chi. In this context, "strong" refers to the ability of the nerves to convey messages between the mind and the chi clearly, with sufficient "insulation" and "resistance" to avoid burnout. A strong nervous system allows messages to be delivered between the brain and the chi without conscious will or effort. Until the nerves have been developed, the will must be used to transmit messages, much as a baby at first has to use tremendous will power to crawl and walk until the appropriate nervous pathways between the brain and the chi are forged. Once those links

are in place, you do not need to think about walking, you simply walk.

The development of chi must of necessity be slow and
steady in order for it to be stable. Once this is understood, it is
easy to see how the incorrect practice of Chi Gung can lead to
problems.

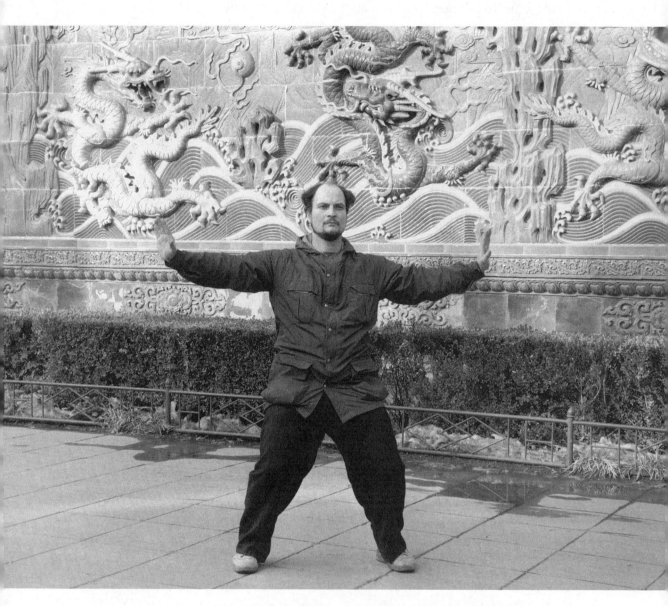

Bruce Kumar Frantzis demonstrates one of the 200 or so Chi Gung standing postures at the Nine Dragon Wall in Beijing, China, in the winter of 1986.

CHAPTER 2

Chi Gung Theory

The Gap between Chi Gung as It Is Taught in China and the West

Since returning from ten years of intense study of the internal arts in China, I have conducted workshops and taught classes attended by many Tai Chi and Chi Gung students and teachers, who had anywhere from one to twenty years of experience. It has been my observation that many of the most fundamental (and essential) principles of Tai Chi and Chi Gung have never been explained to these individuals, many of whom are now, or will be, teachers of these arts.

In fact, at the present time, much of the Western practice of the internal arts (Tai Chi Chuan, Chi Gung, Nei Gung, Hsing I Chuan, and Ba Gua Chang; see p. 7), is based solely on physical movements and mental visualizations. Many students only imitate the external movements of their teachers, believing that this type of practice will increase their flow of chi, thereby giving them power and health. These students have to guess at what their teachers are doing internally, with no way of knowing if their guesses are correct.

The Challenge of the Chinese Language Barrier

Other students whom I have taught did receive explanations about internal energy from their Chinese teachers; unfortunately, the information imparted was not always accurate, as their teachers often did not speak English well and the translators lacked sufficient knowledge to translate this highly technical subject into English. Vague generalities were often substituted for specific information. In many cases, the problem was the original teacher's sheer *unwillingness* to transmit the specific training methodologies clearly.

In the process of transferring wisdom from one culture to another, difficulties and common misunderstandings are the rule rather than the exception. Now that Tai Chi and Chi Gung have been known in the West for twenty or thirty years, the time has come to help clear up people's misconceptions about these arts.

A majority of the early translators were not themselves expert in the fields of Tai Chi and Chi Gung. Consequently, metaphorical descriptions were commonly mistaken for actual methods of practice. As in any specialized field, technical terms can have radically different meanings and connotations for insiders. The general public may be familiar with the words themselves, but be ignorant of their precise intent. Since most people with expertise in the field of chi development are Chinese, metaphors in the Chinese language are used to describe what adepts are doing. These metaphors make perfect sense from an Oriental perspective, but often lead Westerners down the wrong path. Of course, this problem also applies in reverse with regard to the transfer of technology from the West to the East; Orientals frequently misinterpret Western ideas about how to do things.

As much as possible, this chapter will try to demystify and clarify the common cross-cultural confusion inherent in this area and, more importantly, will convey in contemporary English the processes that are involved in the basic practices of these internal arts.

The Challenge of Transplanting Chinese Cultural Ideas

After I became truly bilingual, I noticed that *even when I'm processing the same information in my mind, I think and feel quite differently in each language*. This happens because the cultural and linguistic context in which people learn to view life determines to a great extent what they feel, and how they think information should be communicated. This cultural matrix dictates not only what *should* remain unstated but also how what was left unsaid should be interpreted.

These issues have caused great difficulties in communicating the subjects of Tai Chi and Chi Gung to Westerners. Orientals leave much unsaid, assuming that much of what is relegated to silence anybody (meaning anyone with an average Oriental education) would understand. Unfortunately, the Oriental cultural background contains information that most Westerners have no access to. Let us, then, begin with some basic definitions.

Traditional Chi Gung and Nei Gung— What's the Difference?

Up until fifty years ago, the term *Chi Gung* was rarely used in China for chi development practices; the more prevailing terms were *Nei Gung* (internal power) and *Lien Gung* (practice power). During the last half century, however, the term *Chi Gung* has gained ascendancy, especially in mainland China, where one finds a variety of forms, many with poetic or strange names, such as White Crane Chi Gung, Old Man Climbs the Stairs Chi Gung, Plum Blossom Chi Gung, and so forth.

All Chi Gung practices are derived from the parent Nei Gung systems. (The techniques found in this volume, for example, are all original Nei Gung practices.*)

Nei Gung Moves from the Inside Out; Chi Gung Moves from the Outside In

The emphasis in Nei Gung is on developing the core energy that travels through the center of the body, and, from the core, opening and energizing the peripheral energy lines (the acupuncture meridians, for example). Chi Gung concentrates on working the more superficial energy lines first, and, through these, affecting the core energy. In this sense, Chi Gung is similar to acupuncture, which also manipulates the more superficial and peripheral energy through the meridians, collateral channels, and eight special meridians to bring about changes at a deeper level.

*Editor's note: Throughout this book, the author uses the term Chi Gung as a kind of brand name that is familiar to the West. The material in this book actually involves Nei Gung practices that are known as Chi Gung in the popular mind.

Chi Gung Moves Chi with a Sequence of Body Movements; Nei Gung Moves Chi through Multiple Mind-Body Interactions

In Chi Gung, the practitioner works one technique at a time, combining them gradually into a specific sequence. For instance, one acupuncture channel is opened, then, once opened, the practitioner opens the next in line, and so on. There are any number of techniques used in Chi Gung, from slapping to stretching to stomping, but the most important principle to remember about Chi Gung in general is that one chi flow is sequentially *followed* by another. Two or more rarely go on simultaneously.

The Nei Gung system, on the other hand, seeks to work all the chi flows of the system at one time, the ultimate objective being to synergistically combine the hundreds of chi flows in the body. This way, the practitioner will eventually have access to energy which, in its totality, is more than just the sum of the chi flowing through the channels. At high levels, the chi of the body, mind, and spirit integrates. The whole person then functions in the manner of a single huge cell, with all its chi pulsing in unison.

Of course, Nei Gung is learned one piece at a time, but it is practiced in a way that all learned pieces are performed simultaneously. Eventually, the practitioner's energy permeates to the center of both the bone marrow and the spine. For this reason, Nei Gung is generally considered superior for people who want to have both superior health and great physical prowess.

Put simply, the main difference between Chi Gung and Nei Gung is that, in Chi Gung, technique A is followed by technique B followed by technique C; the effect of these is the cumulative effect of A plus B plus C. With Nei Gung, however, technique A is done at the same time as B and C; synergistically, the effect is that of A multiplied by B multiplied by C.

In Chi Gung, the Breath Is a Vehicle for the Movement of Chi; in Nei Gung, the Mind Moves the Chi Directly

In the Chinese internal arts, the term "breath" refers to two distinct processes: first, the movement of air in and out of the lungs, which we will call the physical oxygen breath; and second, the ebb and flow of the chi or life force throughout the body, which we will call the subtle breath. The physical breath and the subtle breath can be coordinated, or they can work independently. Chi Gung coordinates the two, while Nei Gung works directly with the subtle breath, without the need for the intermediary of the physical breath.

In Chi Gung, the physical breath is used to forge a link between the mind and the chi or subtle breath. The mind or awareness focuses on the physical breath: you visualize the physical breath moving chi through your body and you feel the breath go into a particular part of your body. It thus makes contact with the chi or subtle breath. The in/out, suspension, and quickening/slowing of the physical breath is coordinated with whatever one is doing, whether it be body movement, energy development, or visualization of the emotional, psychic, or spiritual aspects of one's being.

Most Chinese medical Chi Gung methods are based on the use of the physical breath to activate the chi. Similarly, most Buddhist Chi Gung practices are based on awareness of the physical breath.* For example, Gautama the Buddha's essential practice (today known as Vipassana) was based upon observing the rise and fall of the physical breath and the sensations in the body. And Tantric Buddhism uses the rhythm of the physical breath as a coordinating medium for mantras and visualizations.

In Nei Gung, however, the mind or awareness moves the chi directly, without the assistance of the physical breath. The mind may remain purely aware of the internal energy, or may direct it to specific tasks and energy channels. Nei Gung uses efficient physical breathing mechanisms that recreate how a baby breathes in the womb, but chi movement is independent of the physical breath, regardless of how you are breathing. The physical breath at times may become so slow, quiet, and still as to seem to disappear. The context of the subtle breath shifts from the physical breath to the presence of the mind itself.

For a person doing chi development that involves physical movement, Nei Gung has one inherent advantage over Chi Gung. This advantage relates to the subconscious mind. Thoughts and emotions create "waves" in the mind. The way one breathes can also control and create these waves, and can cause the mind to take on the thought wave pattern of specific emotions. For example, when you get angry, your breath rises

*Editor's Note: Mr. Frantzis is at work on a book about Dragon and Tiger Chi Gung, a very effective Buddhist Chi Gung method widely used for Chi Gung cancer therapy in China.

to your chest, and then to your head with short, powerful bursts. Conversely, if you start breathing from the chest and head intentionally with short, powerful bursts, you will start feeling angry. On the other hand, if you are feeling depressed, which usually results in very shallow breathing, and you consciously start deep, regular breathing, you will feel less depressed. You can change or at least mask your feelings with your breath.

Usually, when the breath and the mind are coordinated, one simply experiences the emotion. However, if you practice the Chi Gung method of coordinating the physical breath with the body's movements, you may cause emotional suppression to occur. You will only become aware of your breath and movement, and not your emotions. The artificial breathing pattern masks awareness of your actual emotions, and at the same time, you strengthen these invisible emotions by your practice. Coordinating breath with movement will increase your physical capacities and charge up your physical chi, but it will also charge up the deeper layers of your being, the emotional and psychic basement where lie the emotions that have been repressed over a lifetime.

Thus, in Chi Gung, there is the possibility that emotional energy may be increased but suppressed. If, for example, individuals practice a breathing pattern that increases anger or depression, they could find themselves becoming extremely explosive or easily depressed without knowing why. The stronger one becomes physically, the more an emotional wreck one becomes. Many people in the sports and martial arts community have suffered on this account: One becomes aware of the physical, but not the emotional (or psychic) level of chi.

In Nei Gung, one works directly with the chi, bypassing, at the beginning levels, the use of the breath to move the chi. The practitioner slowly over time becomes sensitive to how the subtle breath or chi is not only penetrating the physical body, but also the more subtle energy bodies—the emotional body, the mental body, psychic body, the causal body, and so on. Once the connection between the mind and the various chi bodies has been stabilized, one will be aware of how the coordination of the breath with physical and chi movement affects all levels of one's being. Such practitioners will then be able to use the breath consciously to develop all of their energy bodies equally. They will become aware of the dark, dead emotional spots that need to be dissolved, as well as the bright, alive spots that should be energized. At this more advanced stage, the use of the breath will allow one to strengthen the whole energy body in a strong and balanced way.

Chi Gung is in general concerned more with specific acupuncture channels and points, whereas Nei Gung works more with the energy running from the crown of the head to the perineum and through the center of the bones of the arms and legs, as well as with the muscles, fascia, internal organs, glands, spinal cord, and brain. From a medical perspective, Chi Gung usually utilizes specific techniques for specific problems, while Nei Gung energizes the whole system, and this overall improvement in energy function leads to the eventual resolution of particular problems.

Chi Gung and Nei Gung Each Have Unique Strengths

As a general rule, a true Nei Gung expert will understand the methodologies of Chi Gung. However, the reverse is not true— a Chi Gung expert will usually not be aware of all the Nei Gung methods. This would lead one to believe that Nei Gung is superior to Chi Gung, which is not necessarily the case. Many diseases and dysfunctions may be caused by an imbalance in only a small part of a person's system. In these cases, it is better to apply Chi Gung techniques because only a limited number of chi flows need to be learned and practiced to address the problem.

The Internal Martial Arts: Tai Chi, Hsing I, and Ba Gua

The three internal martial arts of Tai Chi, Hsing I, and Ba Gua are all based on the Nei Gung system of chi development. They combine the most effective fighting techniques of ancient China and fuse them with the Nei Gung system of internal power development. This combination produces two seemingly unrelated results: superior competitive athletic and fighting skills and superior health. These arts are also, at high levels, complete spiritual development systems.

Tai Chi Is Primarily Practiced for Health in China

In modern China, almost all of the people who practice Tai Chi do so purely to enhance their health, reduce stress, and improve their energy. Relatively few of them use it as a martial art, where the increased internal power is utilized to improve fighting ability, whether for attacking, defending, hitting, or absorbing blows. It should be stressed that the training for martial applications is appreciably more rigorous than that for health. Jogging a mile or two a day may be good for health, but to become a marathoner requires significantly more effort. Similarly, practicing Tai Chi for only 20 to 40 minutes a day can greatly improve well-being, and extend vibrant health into old age, but hours a day are required to become a martial artist. To use Tai Chi to become spiritually realized requires even more effort than martial art training.

Hsing I and Ba Gua: Fighting Methods That Promote Long Life

Hsing I is an extremely powerful Nei Gung system, and has been the main internal system used on battlefields in China for the past nine hundred years. Invented by a general who then taught it to his officer corps, Hsing I, in the nineteenth century, became famous as the martial art of convoy guards. It can be considered like karate with internal power.

As well as producing health, Hsing I places great emphasis on developing strength. While a Tai Chi master's body becomes soft on the outside and hard on the inside, Hsing I masters seek just the opposite. The outside becomes like a piece of steel and the inside becomes very soft, which leads to incredible physical flexibility as well as a sense of internal comfort. Of the three internal martial arts, Hsing I brings a sense of strength and vitality the most quickly.

Ba Gua is generally considered the highest of the internal martial arts. Like Hsing I masters, Ba Gua masters tend to live longer than Tai Chi masters. Ba Gua practices are more difficult than those of Tai Chi. In China, they say that everybody can do Tai Chi, but only a few can do Hsing I and fewer still Ba Gua. Tai Chi and Hsing I use circles, but Ba Gua is unique in its use of spheres. Ba Gua works the energy of the body in such a way that it eventually creates more physical and energetic flexibility than either of the other two internal arts. It is also the most physically beautiful, with its continually manifesting spiraling energy.

While Ba Gua is a very effective martial art, this is but one of its aspects. Based on the energy internal alchemy principles of the *I Ching*, or Book of Changes, Ba Gua is a physical method of embodying and manifesting the *I Ching*'s energies. It is a sad fact that the genuine energy tradition of Ba Gua is being lost in China and the West. Mostly what one can find now of Ba Gua consists of a series of physical movements or simple martial art applications used in diverse martial art schools. It is very difficult to locate substantial information about the genuine Ba Gua system.

Ba Gua is the only martial art in China that is completely Taoist in nature, as both Tai Chi and Hsing I were influenced by the Buddhist Shaolin Monastery. Ba Gua only surfaced about one hundred years ago, though there is a Taoist monastery in southern China that has been practicing the basic Ba Gua walk for 1500 years, and they have records of it coming 4000 years ago from somewhere in the Kunlun mountains. No one really knows how old it is.

The practice sets of all three internal martial arts are composed of a series of postures. In the fashion of all Nei Gung practices, each of these postures works all the body's chi flows simultaneously. As with Chi Gung practices, each Nei Gung posture in the internal arts (whether martial art or Taoist yoga) has one major energetic function, and the entire set is a series of consecutive interlinked postures, each developing a specific energy. The postures done in sequence simultaneously create a Nei Gung-Chi Gung set, with the purpose of clearing blockages, making the overall chi in the body more powerful, and balancing the body's energy system.

The same life energy developed and used by martial artists can also be used by athletes or dancers, enabling them to develop a reserve of inner power that normally only the most talented of champions ever acquire. The difference is that, in the West, athletes find this inner power by accident or birth, whereas the Chinese have found many deliberate, systematic ways of developing this internal power for those willing to take the time to practice consistently.

Three Levels of Chi Gung: Body, Chi, and Mind

The internal methodologies of Tai Chi Chuan, Hsing I Chuan, and Ba Gua Chang, as well as Chi Gung and Nei Gung, all operate on three levels. These may be identified as: (1) technique, (2) mechanics, and (3) technology; or, to put it more concretely, what you do with your body, chi, and mind/spirit at any given point in time.

The core exercises presented in this volume deal primarily with body and chi development. They are not especially concerned with emptying the mind and attaining stillness and union with the Tao, which are goals of higher-level mind development techniques. Before running, one must first learn to stand and walk.

The core exercises herein can have a dual function: (1) you can do them independently, as a form of Chi Gung, even if you know nothing about Tai Chi. Such practice will provide you with many of the basic health and stress-management benefits that motivate most people to begin Tai Chi or other internal martial arts in the first place; (2) If you are already involved in the internal martial arts or in sitting meditation, you can do these exercises as warm-ups, so that your internal organs are fully prepared for practice. Such use reduces the possibility of injuries and dissipates the initial layer of stress that would otherwise have to be dissolved during the first half hour of your regular practice. You are thereby freed to concentrate on the deeper elements of Tai Chi or meditation. Let's take a closer look at the warm-up function.

Chi Gung as an Internal Warm-Up

Used as warm-ups, the core exercises are similar to the warm-ups athletes perform before beginning their respective sports. The Chi Gung exercises are, however, quite unlike the leg stretches and other movements that a runner or karate practitioner performs. Rather, the function of the Chi Gung warm-up is to:

1. make the mind as still, quiet, and stable as possible;
2. bring all the internal connections between the various body parts and the mind into operation;
3. raise the efficiency of internal organs up to a high level;
4. open up the spine and all the joints of the body;
5. promote healing and prevent injuries by increasing awareness of body limitations on any given day.

All of the above is accomplished through internal concentration and motions that are externally small, but internally large, meaning that—from the point of view of someone watching—the practitioner's body may seem to be making small, meaningless motions. Internally, however, dramatic (or "large") events are happening: tissues are expanding and contracting, there is greater control over joint movements, nerve flow is increased, internal organs are pressurized and massaged, conscious awareness of internal body functions is markedly increased—even the fluids that make your body work can be felt and their pumping action increased. If you do these Core Exercises over a long period of time, you can develop a relaxed power and flexibility usually unobtainable by the average person.

Tai Chi, Hsing I Chuan, and Ba Gua Chang are, for many people, too complex and time-consuming to undertake, and the apparent complexity of the movements leads many to become discouraged and quit. These simple exercises have the great advantage, as do all basic Chi Gung and Nei Gung techniques, of having very few external motions, thus allowing the student to devote much more time and energy to internal development. When learned well and practiced diligently, these Core Exercises allow the internal martial arts to be learned much faster and with less frustration.

Chi Gung Improves Body-Mind Connections

There is a great difference between intellectually understanding a physical movement and being able to perform the action. The brain controls the muscles via the nervous system. Some people, especially natural athletes, have marvelously developed nervous systems, and they need only be shown a movement to be able to do it. However, such people are a minority of the population. Also, the speed and facility with which the nervous system learns decreases with age for the average human being. A ten-year-old will learn any athletic function much more rapidly than someone forty or fifty.

Fortunately, the ancient Chinese Taoists developed ways to train the nervous system to better link the mind and body, and they took this knowledge further than any other culture. Just as there is no need to re-invent the wheel every week, much needless struggle can be avoided by using these ancient techniques to train the nervous system. They can make life in the modern world more comfortable internally, which is a value especially appealing to people over thirty who are at the stage of life where career and family stresses can intensify.

Body Synergy Increases Your Reservoir of Chi

The primary idea behind these core exercises (and, for that matter, behind Tai Chi and Nei Gung in general) is synergy, meaning that the whole can be much more than the sum of the parts. In human activity, synergy is verified experientially. You have to feel it to know whether or not it works. Hundreds of millions of people throughout the centuries in China, and many people in the West, have found that using energy synergistically is of great value.

Simply put, synergy in the core exercises involves coordinating the many elements of body, mind, and energy so that they move simultaneously. For example, if five parts of your body, each having an arbitrary value of two, were to work separately or consecutively (as they would for most people), the resulting energy would be equal to the sum of the parts, or 10 units. Using the parts synergistically would be like multiplying the energy values of the parts, rather than just adding them, and the energy output would equal 32 units.

All of these exercises are performed with the intention of strengthening the central nervous system and the internal organs, rather than only the muscles. Through the application of total relaxation, they first seek to rid the body of accumulated stress and tension. Next, they strengthen the internal organs and nerves of the body, as much as the practitioner's capacity allows. When this capacity is reached, they then increase reserves that can be drawn on naturally in times of stress or emergency.

From the perspective of chi development, many exercises done in the West have a tendency to deplete the body's essential core reserves, mainly because they are so performance-oriented. The competition may be won today, but ten or fifteen years down the road, when deep reserve energy is needed to fight off internal organ problems or cancer, it will not be there. As the adage goes, "the follies of youth are paid for in old age."

The Importance of Preserving Your "Life Capital"

Chi Gung practitioners in China believe that a person is born with a certain amount of life (energy) capital. Let's say most people come into the world with a million dollars, though some rare individuals may be born with hundreds of millions of dollars. For babies, the difference isn't that great between having capital of a million dollars or a hundred million dollars—almost all babies are relaxed, amazingly energetic, and able to recover from illness or injury quickly and easily. (It's like a very rich man who isn't much affected economically whether he eats at McDonalds or the Ritz—for him, there isn't much difference between two dollars and two hundred dollars.) The multimillionaires, because of their tremendous genetic good fortune, can smoke three packs of cigarettes and drink two bottles of whisky a day, cavort into the late hours of the night, get next to no sleep, work inhumanely long hours, and still live to be ninety-five years old without serious illness. For the other 99.9% of the population, however, a lifestyle like this would cause great misery and an early demise.

Major illnesses or injuries or major surgery deplete one's life-energy capital significantly. One either makes up this capital or lives diminished until death. Chi Gung can replace this lost energy, enabling people to make up any deficit and recover normal living.

Your Core Reserve of Energy Is Critical

Obviously, through eating nutritional food, getting appropriate exercise, and living moderately, one can generate a certain amount of life-energy that can be used on a day-to-day basis, improving general well-being. Unfortunately, this regimen may not add to the *core* reserves, and one must realize that prolonged stress can burn up core reserves so rapidly that illness may occur. Core reserves are meant for emergencies and disasters, not for daily activities.

The person who lives intelligently will have more than the average energy reserves left to help recover from hard times, but the person who increases core reserves can go from being poor to being rich. This increase in internal wealth, unlike material wealth, cannot be taxed or stolen. And it cannot come from manipulating other people's capital—it must be earned.

When a person's reserves increase significantly, most of the aches and pains, tensions, and general physical discomforts of life vanish. The practice of these core exercises (or Tai Chi) is a direct investment in the future, just as small daily investments of money compounded lead to large sums down the road. Herein is not the path of instant gratification, though almost immediately there will be a sense of increased well-being and body ease. The real value of these exercises will become obvious as the years go on, as the energy or capital gained grows ever larger.

Chi Gung's Fundamental Principle: Heaven, Earth, and Man

All Tai Chi Chuan practices, as well as those of Chi Gung, are based on the fundamental Chinese concepts of Heaven, Earth, and Man (Tien, Di, Ren). Energy from the Earth is drawn upward from the practitioner's root; the root being slightly below the spot where the foot touches the earth. Energy descends from Heaven through the crown of the head. We are in the middle, and need to receive energy from both of these sources, which in effect are like positive and negative poles. When the positive and negative are connected, the life current can flow naturally. This current can be used on a day-to-day basis, and with training it can be stored in the body like electricity is stored in a car battery.

The Components of Standing

Posture

The first component of standing concerns the physical alignment of the body. If the body parts are not properly aligned, energy will leak out or dam up, as water would in a poorly constructed plumbing system. Most of the places where these blockages or leakages first occur in the human body are in and around the joints.

The Descending Chi Current: From Heaven to Earth

The second component involves bringing energy from Heaven through the body and down to Earth, which is purely an energetic process. A fundamental principle of Chi Gung and Nei Gung training, unfamiliar to most people in the West, is that the energy moving from above to below is basically responsible for general well-being.

The energetic system in the human body is a bit like an electrical system. Before power can be put through a wire, the system must have the correct insulation and resistance. If such is not the case, the system can burn out or short circuit. From the Chinese point of view (or from the Indian yogic viewpoint), it is not all that difficult to develop plenty of energy. The difficulty lies in creating a system strong enough to use this current, rather than be damaged by it. Therefore, much of the beginner's time is spent developing the safety measures and internal resistance necessary to ensure that the system is not damaged by adding too much energy too quickly.

This consideration means that in any Chi Gung or Nei Gung practice, before energy is sent through specific circuits, the body's capacity to withstand the increased current must be developed. The greater the amount of power to be put through an electrical system, the thicker the wires, the heavier the insulation, and the stronger the fuses needed.

In Chi Gung and Nei Gung, the system's capacity is increased by developing the downward current of energy. This clears out blockages and strengthens the ability of the central nervous system to hold energy when the current rises upward. Therefore, in the beginning, a much greater proportion of time and practice is spent on grounding energy than on raising it.

Many people experience involuntary shaking when standing. This shaking is symptomatic of bound physical or emotional energy releasing from the body. This is the same situation that often occurs when someone is getting an acupuncture treatment—the release of bound energy can make your body vibrate rather than the needle. Commonly, however, when an acupuncture needle is inserted into a blocked acupuncture point, the blocked energy grabs the needle and vibrates it. Once the energy blockage is removed, the needle ceases to vibrate because the acupuncture meridian opens.

As energy blocks are cleared by the downward current, energy that has been blocked in the body for long periods of time is freed up, and the body can use this energy easily and comfortably. The only general symptoms that can be disconcerting here are those that occur after the clearing out of very strong blockages. In such instances, there will be a temporary feeling of strong fatigue, as toxins are released from the body and the body undergoes a transition from a lower to a higher energy level. This should not be a source of concern, and it is generally considered a sign of progress. Once this transition is complete, the practitioner will have more energy and vitality than before.

The Ascending Chi Current: From Earth to Heaven

The third phase involves bringing energy up the body, from below the ground to above the head, or from Earth to Heaven. In many schools of energetics, this is the current that is emphasized, primarily because of its spiritualizing effects. This is the phase where people tend to begin having "spiritual experiences," such as psychic experiences, visions, internal sounds, and out of body experiences as well as, to be honest, all manners of hallucinations, spacing out, and general disassociation from the body.

When energy is flowing evenly, powerfully, and naturally through you, you will experience a sense of comfort, ease, and relaxed clarity. It is blockages that create sensations. These experiences can seem to be either positive or negative. What needs to be understood about them is that they are all just essentially experiences of energy blockages. If the blockage feels bad, a person wants to "work through it," and a sense of achievement comes from emptying the garbage.

Lights, sounds, visions, and other psychic phenomena are assumed to be great boons, to be coveted and possessed at all costs. The classic hook used to control people in all sorts of manipulative energy practices involves getting them to think that they are special, or more powerful or elevated than other people, simply because they have these paranormal experiences and can project energy in odd or unusual ways. This can easily lead people to substitute these psychic experiences for alcohol, cocaine, and other addictive substances, in effect creating an energy junkie. Although this form of energy work is a much more positive addiction than drugs or other obsessive behaviors, it still is not the true intent of these exercises.

The sense of well-being and clarity that comes when energy is flowing smoothly does not have the incredible power surges and larger-than-life quality to it that many imagine. It is, rather, just a very natural ease and connectedness to oneself, to one's normal interactions in life, and to one's physical, mental, and spiritual bodies. When the shoe truly fits the foot, the shoe is forgotten, and one just walks, easily and comfortably.

Humans Must Balance These Currents

In the Chinese internal energy practices, eight units of time and effort are usually spent in developing the descending current and two units of time and effort in developing the ascending current, so that all the safety precautions are in place before too much juice is put in the system. Many people throughout history, in many countries and traditions, have concentrated almost exclusively on the upward current, and a tremendous amount of unnecessary burnout has been the result. (See Appendix C for further information.)

The Chinese realize that energy is always around and has always existed, and through the power of the mind its form can be changed greatly. The mind, through its capacity to project, is able to direct the chi, using the medium of the central nervous system. Chi is bound with blood in the human body, and this chi-infused blood has the ability to reach every cell of the body. The connection between the mind and chi is the nerves. The nerves play a critical role in Chi Gung practice, and are the metaphorical wiring that we discussed before. It is through the transformation of the nerves, the actual physical nerves, that the chi can be directed by the mind.

The nerves of the human body take longer to develop than almost any other tissue, and once developed they do not change as rapidly as other tissues. This means that the longer and more steadily Chi Gung is practiced, the more permanent and long lasting the effects will be. Chi Gung works to permanently change the nervous system with slow, steady practice.

Do Not Skip Steps in Chi Gung Training

While there is a fair amount of theory included in the material herein, this volume primarily teaches the practical application of many principles of Chi Gung. It is meant to be used as a workbook. Consequently, the movements are presented in sequence, step by step, with suggestions about how much time to spend on each. Each piece builds upon the previous one, and you must let an individual step stabilize (that is, be able to do it with ease) before you move on to the next. If you jump ahead in your practice, you may, besides wasting your time, find yourself creating a weakness in your energy structure, and it often takes four or five times as long to correct this kind of weakness as it took to acquire it. Therefore, take your time, and for maximum benefit do not leap ahead in doing these motions, even out of curiosity, but work with each movement as it comes up. If you merely want to satisfy your intellectual curiosity, *reading* ahead will not matter, but if you want this material to manifest practically in your life, you must physically practice it in sequence.

The human mind is capable of receiving a tremendous amount of information simultaneously. However, there is a world of difference between receiving something and being able to assimilate and use it. Scientific studies indicate that the human mind can only assimilate approximately seven "bits" of information at any given time before it overloads and basically scrambles the information. In Chi Gung, the mind is asked to understand and co-ordinate the material, and the tissue and nerves to remember it.

Chi Gung requires both intellectual and physical comprehension. The kinesthetic sense of balance, energy, and internal body activities is significantly more difficult to learn than the intellectual information. A Ph.D. cannot assume that his mental capacities will help him to play the game of handball faster than someone of a lesser scholastic level. *No matter who you are*, Chi Gung must be learned slowly and gradually. There is no reason to feel anxious if you progress at a rate that seems slower than that of those around you.

Digest Your Chi Slowly, with Frequent Repetition

After twenty years of teaching these movements to large numbers of people of varying ages, physical capacities, and intellectual talents, I have found that the way people learn Chi Gung best is through deliberate repetition. When things were not deliberately repeated over and over again in classes, people stated that they understood, but in fact did not.

So, take your time, and follow instructions carefully. I would not say that Chi Gung is easy to learn, but I would say that it is not all that difficult, especially when you consider its incredible benefits.

The Core Exercises

The Core Exercises in this book are composed of six primary parts. The first is the basic Nei Gung standing posture, and the second is Cloud Hands, which integrates the internal principles learned in the standing postures into the movement of the body as one coordinated synergistic whole. Here, one also learns the essential coordination of the hand movements of Tai Chi. The next three elements are swing movements, which primarily function to open the joints of the arms and legs and infuse the internal organs with energy. The sixth part is a spinal stretch, quite unlike any other, which has the primary function of gaining control of each and every vertebra of the spine and its related nerve and chi flow.

Let us now turn to actually learning the movements.

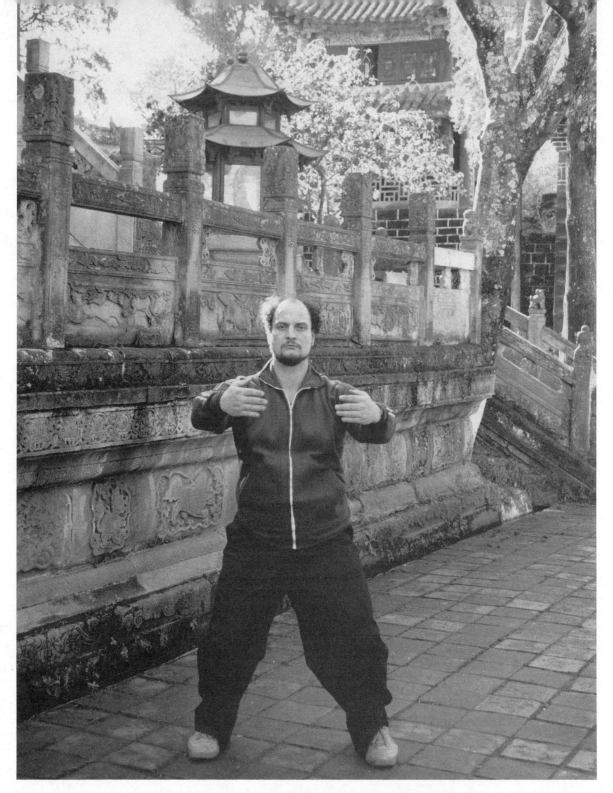

The author demonstrates a basic Chi Gung standing posture at a temple in Kunming, China, in January 1987.

g Posture:

g Body,

Mind

The standing posture (see Fig. 3-1), called *Jan Juang* or "stand strong," is a powerful meditation used to develop internal power. Some Chi Gung masters use this method alone as their daily practice. It is fundamental to Chi Gung, Nei Gung, and Tai Chi Chuan, as it opens the energy gates of the body and so allows the free movement of chi. The techniques of standing are described in a series of sequential lessons, and the material in each lesson must be practiced and understood before moving on to the next. Both body and energy mechanics are discussed in each lesson. The third lesson involves the internal dissolving process, which is explained in easily understood terms.

Lesson One: Body Mechanics

Placement of the Feet

▶ **Your Stance Must Be Comfortable**

Begin standing with the outer edges of your feet somewhere between hip and shoulder width apart, wherever you find it to be most stable and comfortable. The appropriate stance will become more obvious with practice and depends on the relationship between the width of the hips and shoulders. A person with wide

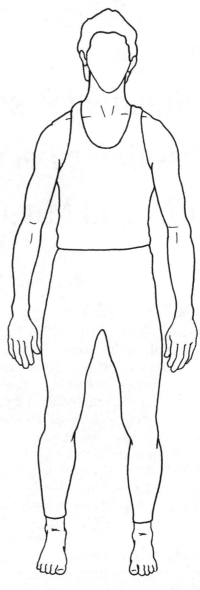

Figure 3-1 Standing posture. Feet are parallel, shoulder-width apart.

shoulders and narrow hips will generally want a stance closer to hip width, while a person with narrow shoulders and wide hips will tend towards a stance closer to shoulder width. Eventually, the center of each foot will align with the left and right energy channels of the body.

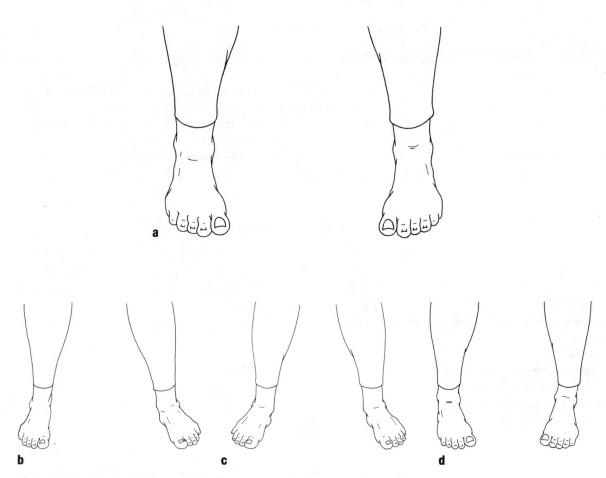

Figure 3-2 (a) Correct: feet parallel. (b) Incorrect: one foot splayed outward. (c) Incorrect: both feet splayed outward. (d) Incorrect: feet turned inward.

▶ Keep Your Feet Parallel to Each Other

The knees should be slightly bent and the feet parallel. Parallel placement of the feet means that the distance between the toes is the same as the distance between the heels, and one foot is neither in front of nor in back of the other (Fig. 3-2a). For example, if the feet are fifteen inches apart, then there should be fifteen inches between the big toes of each foot and fifteen inches between the heels of each foot and each knee.

Placement of the Spine

▶ Your Tailbone Should Point to the Ground

Your tailbone should be perpendicular to the floor (Fig. 3-3a); it should not point backward, as it does when you stand normally. The lower back, from the tailbone up to and including the lumbar vertebrae, must be absolutely straight. In most people, the spine naturally has an "S" shape, with curves at the bottom, middle, and top. In the standing posture discussed here, however, the lower part of the spine is straightened.

▶ Gently Straighten Your Spine

Your spine should be straightened by (1) gently rolling the hips under, and (2) using the inner back muscles to push the kidneys slightly back. Together, these two processes will make the lower part of the spine totally straight.

Figure 3-3 (a) Correct: lower back straight, perpendicular to the floor. (b) Incorrect: lower back curved, buttocks protruding.

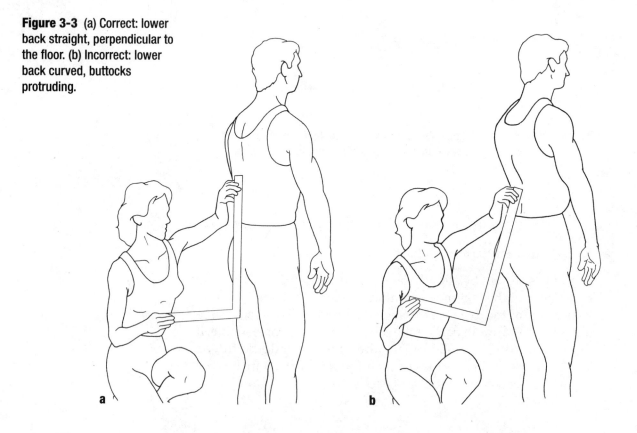

a   b

Obviously, human beings come in various and sundry sizes. For those of thin or medium build, the easiest way to determine if the back is straight is to check if the buttocks are protruding backwards. If this is the case, the posture is not correct. For those having heavier builds, the buttocks may give the impression that the back is swayed even when the back is in fact straight. For this type of physique, the important point is that the back and sacrum are straight, and not whether the buttocks stick out.

As for the rest of the back, it should be kept fairly straight, and should not lean in any direction.

Placement of the Neck and Head

▶ **Your Head Should Float Lightly Above
Your Neck, Which Is Held Straight**

The neck and head need to be held straight (Fig. 3-4a); the crown of the head faces straight up so that a line drawn straight up from the crown would be perpendicular to the ground. As the neck and shoulders relax, quite commonly the head will want to tilt. It is preferable that the head remain upright, but a slight forward tilt is acceptable. Also, it is important to gently lift the occiput from the atlas vertebra (that is, lift the skull gently off the neck bone) to reduce compression of the neck vertebrae. The Chinese liken this to the feeling of lifting a hat off a coatrack.

This essential element of Chi Gung, which will hold true for all movements of the Core Exercises, is called *ding*, or raising the head. *Ding* stretches the spinal cord of the neck area, making sure that the weight of the skull (1) does not compress or misalign the vertebrae of the neck and (2) does not close down the flow of chi and/or nerve energy from the hind brain to the spinal cord. Such closure occurs if pressure is brought to bear on the atlas/axis, the last vertebra at the base of the skull. This principle of *ding* must be present during all standing, moving, or sitting Chi Gung practices. To do this, first hold the neck completely vertical. The jaw is then drawn slightly back, so that the eyes and jaw are exactly parallel to the ground and the crown of the skull moves vertically upwards. This action stretches the vertebrae of the neck and lifts the skull slightly. It must not be done in such a way as to create any tension or stiffness in the jaw, neck, head, or shoulders.

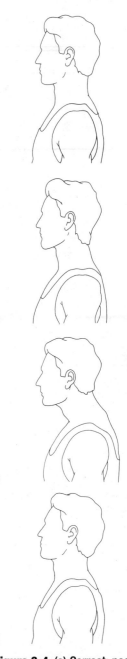

a

b

c

d

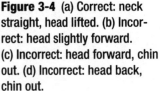

Figure 3-4 (a) Correct: neck straight, head lifted. (b) Incorrect: head slightly forward. (c) Incorrect: head forward, chin out. (d) Incorrect: head back, chin out.

The Eyes and the Tongue

▶ **Beginners Practice with Eyes Shut;
Tongue Touches Roof of Mouth**

In standing, your eyes should be kept initially closed to facilitate your going inward. There are many practices where the eyes remain open, but these are not recommended for beginners. Beginners usually need all of their concentration to keep track of everything that is occurring internally, without attending to the external environment. (Another volume of this series—*The Spiraling Energy Body*—will present advanced practices that enable people—with their eyes open—to dissolve the influence of external stimuli in the same way that they clear out energy blockages internally.)

The tongue should be kept touching the roof of the mouth during all Chi Gung practices, the tip of the tongue should be held against the roof of the mouth. This action is necessary in order to complete the microcosmic circulation of energy in the body. The point on the roof of the mouth is where the major yang and yin energies of the body meet.

Placement of the Chest

▶ **Gently Allow Your Chest to Sink as It Rounds**

Han shiung ba bei, or "round the chest and raise the spine" is a fundamental technique found in all Taoist meditation, internal martial arts, and Chi Gung practices, regardless of school. *Han shiung* means to have a half chest, or chest like an hour glass: that is, it is rounded on both the vertical and horizontal planes. This is like the posture of a baby, where the chest is very relaxed, the shoulders are relaxed downward, and the belly is rounded, dropped, and popped out like that of a sumo wrestler (Fig. 3-5a). The standard western military pose, with the chest thrown out, stomach in, and shoulders and buttocks pushed back, is the exact opposite of this.

▶ **Your Chest Should Expand Toward
Your Navel and the Sides of Your Ribs**

It is very important to understand that in no way, shape, or form do you collapse or depress the chest. This will simply cause the

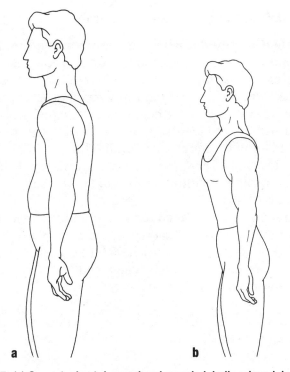

a   b

Figure 3-5 (a) Correct: chest dropped and rounded, belly relaxed, back straight.
(b) Incorrect: chest out, belly tensed, back arched.

lungs to be compressed. In dropping the chest, it remains relaxed
so that, from the inside edge of the shoulders (below the end of
the collarbone—what the Chinese call the shoulder's nest) all the
way through the belly to the hips, there is a sense of sinking,
dropping, and opening downwards. On the side, there is a sense
of the chest and ribs softening and spreading, allowing the chest
to attain its full size without being compressed.

This is based on the principle that the *tantien*, the area in
the lower abdomen where chi is stored, is like a reservoir or
bowl, and that by relaxing the chest downwards, the chi will
drop from the upper body and collect in the lower *tantien*. If the
chest is raised up, the chi will rise upwards rather than sink,
which commonly will result in an angry or overly forceful or
aggressive disposition. In the external martial arts this is called *ti
shiung*, which means "raising the chest." *Ti shiung* creates the
classic V-shaped body, with overdeveloped chest and arm
muscles.

▶ Your Chest Should Stay as Soft as a Baby's

Han Shiung (the rounded chest) is based on the fundamental Taoist proposition that one should make one's body like that of a child, as children are totally natural, unconditioned beings, and as such are wonderfully and naturally efficient. Children, especially babies before they have begun to imitate their elders, have big bellies and relaxed chests. For their size, babies are stronger and more filled with energy than adults. Try to feel the strength a child has for its size, and how relaxed it is. Also, note how they can scream for hours without any trouble. Most adults can not keep up with a baby.

The Taoists found that children and animals (also not conditioned) have something in common. Both breathe from the belly and have a relaxed chest, such that the internal organs drop downward and are massaged by each breath and movement of the body. Observe cats or dogs, cows or horses, and see how their bellies swing from side to side as they walk. This "squashing" of the internal organs strengthens them, in much the same way that massage makes the muscles of the body healthier and stronger.

▶ Give Your Organs an Internal Massage

Gladiators in ancient Rome were massaged every day during training and especially in the mornings before a contest so that they might give a good show. The same effect can be brought about through this relaxing of the chest and dropping of the internal organs. In the classic V-shaped body, the internal organs are pulled up, placing them in fairly fixed positions, which segment the body into upper, middle, and lower thirds. This reduces internal pressure and causes the internal organs to receive a minimum of massage through breathing and movement.

Internal pressure is extremely important, in that it causes the endocrine system and the glands of the body to maximize their secretions. A similar internal pressure is created in hatha yoga (which also develops the classic "V" shape body). In hatha yoga, however, rather than all the endocrine glands of the system being affected simultaneously, specific exercises exist for each gland. In standing postures and Nei Gung work in general, all systems are worked simultaneously. The end result of this relaxation of the chest is to allow energy to drop to the *tantien*, where it is stored like money in a great body bank account, to be used as necessary.

▶ Raise Your Spine and Spread Your Shoulder Blades

Ba bei refers to the raising of the spine. The lungs need to expand and open in order to breathe. In the V-shape body practices, the chest is pushed forward (convex), and the back arched as the shoulder blades raise up and converge towards the spine. Conversely, in the raising of the spine (back), for Nei Gung two things occur.

First, the spine physically raises up, as if it were being pulled upwards. This takes the curve out of the upper back. The term *ba* in Chinese means to pluck something up, like pulling grass or a plant out of the ground. So as the chest is moving downwards, the back and spine are raising upwards, which allows the lungs plenty of room on a vertical plane.

Second, on the horizontal plane, the back becomes totally rounded (Fig. 3-6a). Instead of the shoulder blades coming together as they do in the military posture, they relax downward, spread as far apart as possible, so that the lungs expand backwards towards the spine. When these two principles are combined with the straightening of the lower back, the net result is a series of yin/yang balances that are the exact opposite of the standard military V-shaped posture.

In the standard military posture, the chest is out, and the rear end has shifted backwards. In the Taoist position, the chest is rounded into a half moon shape, and the back is flat with the pelvis tilting forward. In the military posture, the stomach is sucked in and the chest raised up, while in the Taoist posture the chest is relaxed downwards and the belly is dropped. In the military posture, the bottom and top of the spine are clearly curved. In the Taoist posture, they are basically straight.

The Taoist posture also makes it easier to breathe naturally from the diaphragm, in the way that opera singers and babies do. Taoists consider this way of breathing to be ideal for adults.

Small Heavenly Orbit: Internal Organs Sink as the Spine Rises

From the pelvis up to the ribs, on the sides of the body (at the midriff), the internal oblique muscles should perform a lifting or raising action to prevent downward compression, which allows the vertebrae of the lower spine to remain straight, with plenty of intervertebral space. This muscular lifting is done simultaneously with the front of the body sinking downwards, so

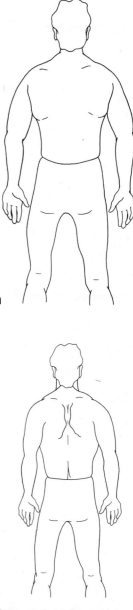

a

b

Figure 3-6 (a) Correct: shoulder blades spread, shoulders rounded forward. (b) Incorrect: shoulder blades drawn toward spine, shoulders pushed back.

that in the trunk of the body, between the solar plexus and the hips, there is a sinking as well as a rising.

The lifting of the spine and the dropping of the internal organs and chi together create the Small Heavenly Orbit of Energy, sometimes called the Microcosmic Orbit or Small Circulation. This is called *shao jyou tien* in Chinese, and has been openly written about and practiced for thousands of years in China.

There *are* deeper, more secretive and esoteric aspects of this practice, however, that *must be learned under the strict guidance of a teacher* to prevent bodily harm. The material in this book regarding the circulation of energy is fairly common knowledge in China among people who do this kind of work, and is quite safe to practice. Some energy practices *are* kept secret because to reveal them to a general audience would be like putting a gun in the hand of a child. Many things are not taught in Chi Gung until a certain amount of experience and maturity is established in the student.

Palms Face Backwards as Hands Rest on the Sides of Your Thighs

This posture is the most energetically neutral pose. It is ideal for beginners practicing standing. This position specifically keeps the armpits open so that the left and right energy channels do not close down.

Lesson Two: Scan Your Energy Body

▶ **Slowly Observe Any Energy Imbalances in Your Body**

While standing in the posture described in Lesson One (Fig. 3-7), scan your body internally from top to bottom. Beginning at the top of your head, start to notice places in your body where you feel any tension, strength, discomfort, or anything that just doesn't feel quite right. Pay special attention to those places where you don't know just what it is that doesn't feel quite right. Feel any sense of contraction or binding. From the top of the head all the way down to the bottom of the feet, explore your body internally millimeter by millimeter, simply taking inventory of what you feel, noticing any spots, no matter how small or how subtle, that reflect the above conditions. Continue this process to below your feet, if possible. If not, it doesn't matter—this ability will come in time. It must be emphasized that you are not to do anything with these sensations; simply become aware, and take inventory of where they are.

Helpful Hints for Awakening Your Chi

▶ **Take Your Time**

Usually it will take from fifteen minutes to an hour to accomplish what we call awakening the chi. If you feel you have accomplished this in two or three minutes you have definitely not done the exercise correctly.

▶ **Internal Scanning Is a Feeling,** *not* **a Visualization Exercise**

In doing your internal review, you may not have directly felt your body, but merely visualized it, which is an infinitely easier task. You may not like some of the things you *did* feel, but these places will not go away if they are buried or ignored—they must be worked through. You need to *allow yourself* to feel the actual state of your insides. You will, over time, gain the power to release your internal blockages.

▶ **Let Your Nerves Come Alive**

One of the main purposes of energy development practices is to promote an entirely new capacity for feeling. The difference in body awareness between a paraplegic and an average person will be as wide as the gap between your present and future state of nerve awareness once your chi practices are established. Don't be frustrated if you can't feel much at first. In time, you *will* be able to feel.

▶ **Keep the Mind Stable**

Energy body scanning is not essentially a physical or an intellectual exercise. It is an exercise in specifying, refining, and increasing the life-force energies in the body. Small children are known for their short attention spans, but most adults also have what the Chinese call a "monkey mind"—a mind that can't stand still and jumps from place to place. The mind of the chi development practitioner, like that of a child, develops slowly.

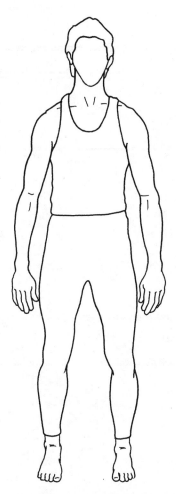

Figure 3-7 Standing posture: feet parallel, spine straight, head lifted, chest dropped, belly relaxed, shoulders rounded.

Gradually, this practice increases your attention span, concentration, and sensitivity to subtle energies.

▶ **The Need for Rapid Perfection Slows Progress**

Again, it must be understood that this is a process of gradual development. Only the rarest of human beings can do these exercises correctly in the beginning. In the practice of chi development, the more gentle and consistent you are, the faster and more steady your progress will be. Mentally or metaphorically whipping yourself on will only result in discouragement, even when you are in fact progressing normally.

▶ **Beware of False Feelings of Strength**

To most people, a sense of strength is a very positive and useful thing, something to be valued and sought after. The weight lifter prizes it as much as an executive at a power lunch or a used car salesman closing a deal. In chi work, however, the feeling of "strength" is considered a blockage. A feeling of strength is found where energy has built up due to blockages, blockages which prevent the normal, healthy, steady, flow of energy from circulating in a relaxed, powerful fashion. The paradox is this: the more you feel your strength, the weaker your chi is. The ideal is for the energy in any given place in the body to feel (1) relaxed, (2) comfortable, with an easy sense of flow, (3) full and balanced, with (4) a total sense of emptiness connected with the energy.

It is only when the energy is blocked that it generates some type of specific feeling. People who grew up with only clean, fresh air wouldn't really notice that the air was clean and fresh. However, if the air became polluted or if they found themselves in a room with very little air, they would soon begin to notice variations in air quality.

Lesson Three: The Chi Dissolving Process

Dissolve Blocked Energy: Ice to Water, Water to Gas

As before, beginning at the crown of your head, notice where you have any feelings of strength, tension, something not being quite right, any general uneasiness, or any sense of contraction. These feelings may be physical, energetic, emotional, or mental.

The blockages giving rise to these sensations must be dissolved. The dissolving process involves feeling as though these places change from ice to water, and from water to gas: from something very dense (ice) to something more dispersed (water), until this "stuff" dissipates outside your body (like gas). Let's take a closer look at this process.

Dissolving: The Transformation of Ice to Water to Gas

Once you have identified a place where your energy is blocked or frozen, producing sensations of strength, tension, discomfort, or contraction, your awareness begins to feel or "see" the outer contours of this frozen energy space. Your awareness then begins to penetrate this solid mass, causing the frozen energy to begin to soften, until you reach the center of the blocked mass. This is the transformation of ice to water. (If you put an ice cube in a pan and heat it on the stove, you will observe that the ice cube melts starting at the outside, and moving slowly toward the center.) Once the entire frozen space in your body becomes soft or flowing (like the water in the pan), you keep your attention on that place and your awareness continues to cause that "water" space to expand until there is a sense of the trapped energy expanding out beyond your body, perhaps as much as a foot or two outside its surface. This is the transformation of water to gas. Like the water in the pan, which will not turn to gas until the ice cube is entirely liquefied, so the dissolving of an energy block moves in stages. The human energy field extends anywhere from six inches to two feet outside the physical body, depending on the strength of the field. This energy field takes negative energy that is leaving the body and recycles it back into the body as neutral energy that the body can then adapt for its needs.

To get a sense of this, clench your fist as tight as you can, until your knuckles turn white, causing your energy to contract. Then put your awareness in your hand and expand your contracted energy until you completely relax your hand (ice to water). Then continue to focus your awareness on your hand until your energy expands out of your hand into the air and your hand feels discorporal, empty of all solidity, with a completely amorphous quality (water to gas).

At the stage of ice-to-water, the body will usually become relaxed, soft, and warm as increased chi flow causes blood circulation to increase. (Remember, the mind moves the chi and the chi moves the blood and other fluids.) At the stage of water-to-gas, pain will disappear and the deepest stresses and discomforts in the body (and, later—in more advanced Chi Gung—in the emotions) will vanish. At the level of ice-to-water, one will feel good, but the root levels of energy blockage will not completely disappear.

At the ice stage, your energy is frozen into a particularly disagreeable shape. At the water stage, the shape becomes fluid, making you feel better temporarily, but the possibility exists for the water to change back into ice. At the gas stage, however, the shape breaks up completely and is recycled back into the body as clean, neutral energy, which adds to one's life energy in a positive way and is then naturally adapted for whatever work is required.

This dissolving technique must be accomplished by feeling it, not by picturing it in your mind's eye. Many people are extremely visual, and, today, visualization techniques are very common. The dissolving process, however, is primarily a kinesthetic or body experience, not a visual one.

The process of ice-to-water-to-gas is more than just a relaxation technique. Relaxation does not necessarily result in more energy, energy that can heal the body. Also, it is possible to relax the muscles and leave emotional blockages untouched. Energetic release affects you on all levels of being.

Standing: Dissolve Downward through the Entire Body

Starting at the crown of your head, dissolve that point or area as completely as possible, until you have an internal sense that it is not possible to dissolve that point or area any further. That is, if you were to continue trying to dissolve that point or area for the next five minutes, five hours, of five years, you would go no further. You then drop whatever energy remains undissolved at the first place down to the next place where energy is bound. You now dissolve this combined energy of the first and second places until you reach again the point of diminishing returns. Drop what remains undissolved down to the third place and again dissolve the combined energies from the first, second, and third places until you again reach the point of diminishing returns, and continue downward, millimeter by millimeter (or inch by inch) to below your feet. Dump everything down to the root of your energy body and into the energy of the earth—release the internal sensations through the soles of your feet into the ground, as far down as your awareness continues.

The Human Energy Body Expands and Contracts

An important point to keep in mind is that, while the human physical body ends at the feet and head, the human energy body extends below the feet and above the head. When a human being reaches full adult size, except under the most unusual circumstances, the physical body size is fixed. However, the size of the energy body, or what some in the West call the aura, can grow or shrink many feet, depending upon the vitality or weakness of a person's internal energy. So, some days you may only be able to get your energy an inch into the ground, and some days you may project it many feet. This fluctuation is absolutely normal until the energy body has been developed and stabilized.

The Principles Behind the Dissolving Process

As recognized both by the ancient Taoists and by modern science, the universe is composed of energies vibrating at different rates. Taoist Chi Gung, a preparation for Taoist internal alchemy, follows the basic alchemical methodology of raising slow, condensed energetic vibrations to more subtle, faster, and expansive vibrations. The experience of the ancient world, including China, has shown that by focusing concentrated attention and awareness on the energetic aspects of one's being, one is able to raise the potential and actual strength of the body, mind, and spirit. This creates physical health, emotional well-being, psychic clarity and abilities, and ultimately leads to the development of one's spiritual nature and ability to become one with the nature of the universe: the Tao.

Be Gentle with Yourself

Don't force your chi. Taoism is the path of gentleness, of flowing water. Don't try to push the river. If you have a block you can't dissolve, go around it and dissolve the rest of your body.

Eventually you'll be able to dissolve it—there's absolutely no rush.

Practice Lesson Three for a minimum of a week or two. Then this practice can be integrated into the next level of the standing Chi Gung, which is called Opening the Energy Gates of the Body.

CHAPTER 4

Opening
the Energy Gates
of the Body

What Are the Energy Gates?

The energy gates are major energy relay stations of the body, where the strength of the life current (chi) moving through the system is regulated. Many gates are located at joints or, more precisely, the actual space between the bones of a joint. Initially, during your standing and dissolving practice, these are the most important places to clear out blockages.

The concept of "energy gates" is not new; rather, it has been passed down to us from ancient China. Originally worked out by Taoists, it has become common to many traditions. However, to the best of my knowledge, it has never been completely described in English.

These gates should not be conceived of as simple anatomical locations. They must be felt with the mind, for they are part of your subtle energy body. From an internal perspective, their locations are approximate and can fluctuate slightly. For acupuncturists, the anatomical location of acupuncture points is valuable, as they utilize these points to put something into the body and use physical markers on the body to get to the approximate location into which a needle is inserted. (The needle indirectly stimulates the body's chi.) Some of the energy gates are the same as the acupuncture points; others are different. The energy gates are like the critical step-up booster stations, each of which controls many smaller power stations. In Chi Gung, on the other hand, the mind is being put directly into the point. You must learn to *feel* these points in order to channel the flow of your chi to stimulate the subtle body to the greatest extent possible. The object is not merely to visualize the gate (though a knowledge of anatomy can help in locating it), but to *feel* the gate precisely so you can learn to increase or decrease the amount of power flowing through the gate, using your will with the same amount of ease with which you can now open or shut your eyes, mouth, or hands. Bear in mind that these gates are inside your body and fluctuate minutely in size, depending on the strength of your chi body. *Consequently, the exact depth inside the body and the exact location of a gate inside your body at a given point in time is not amenable to visual analysis.* The physical and energetic bodies are not identical in form and function, though a good Chi Gung practitioner can feel these energy-gate points in the same manner that other people feel acupuncture needles in their skin. In fact, Chi Gung masters can feel these points in other people as well.

Generally speaking, when we practice "opening" the gates, we will do so in the order given below. Be aware, though, that this order is not written in stone. The most important aspect to remember is that energy and internal sensations always travel *down* the body during the releasing (dissolving) process. The next section explains the locations of the gates to be dissolved.

Important Major and Minor Gates of the Body

When you actually practice the dissolving process, you do not work your way skipping from point to point, energy gate to energy gate, as presented in this book. Rather, you dissolve downwards from the top to the bottom of your body (front, back, and sides simultaneously). The energy gates are points where special attention must be paid as your awareness descends through your body, but anything that is blocked between the energy gates is important and also must be dissolved before moving downward to the next gate. Imagine a great sheet of water descending from the top of your body downwards, dissolving everything in its path. This is how the dissolving process works. This universal energy naturally descends on us every moment, the question is whether or not we can make use of it. This descending "water" is the best defense against burnout from the ascending energy or "fire" that emanates from the earth, and which is prized by many spiritual traditions.

The Head and Neck

In the beginning, for all the gates of the head, the dissolving process should only reach a depth of one-half inch, thereby avoiding the brain. There is a very specific methodology for brain Chi Gung, and it is not a subject for beginners—it should only be studied under the direct supervision of a master.* After a month or two of practice it is permissible to dissolve the entire brain at once, but do not dissolve points in the brain separately.

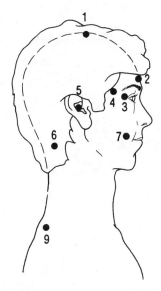

Figure 4-1 Gates of the head and neck.

▶ **(1) The Crown**

The first gate** to be dissolved (see Chapter 3 to review the dissolving process) is at the exact center of the crown of the head, which the Chinese call *bai hwei*, or the "meeting of a hundred points." A line drawn over the head from the nose to the cervical spine (neck) would intersect another line drawn from the apex of one ear to the apex of the other at this point.

▶ **(2) The Third Eye**

Located between the two eyebrows, this point is called the third eye. A person with a history of mental illness should not dissolve this point unless under the supervision of a master. (This gate can open up suppressed areas of a person's psyche, which is best done under the guidance of a qualified master versed in the subtleties of the psychic realm.)

▶ **(3) The Eyes**

This gate is found directly in line with the pupil, just behind the eyeball. This gate is very important for people involved in visually demanding jobs, such as computer operators, as it controls the chi of the visual apparatus and is the interface with the brain. This gate can greatly reduce stress that is visually induced.

▶ **(4) The Center of the Temples**

Usually located on a line from the top of the ear.

*Specific points in the brain may be felt in Chi Gung practice. Connecting these points energetically in certain configurations can be quite dangerous and can cause serious damage to the brain; other connective configurations can enhance the latent powers of the mind. It takes a master with the appropriate knowledge to guide one in this practice.

**Remember that the locations of the gates are approximate. The *exact* locations are to be found by feeling inside your body with your mind.

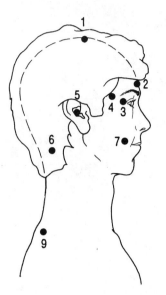

Gates of the head and neck.

▶ **(5) The Center of the Ears**

The next gate is in the center of the ear, no more than one-quarter of the way into the inner ear. (Except for points along the body's center line, all gates are found on both sides of the body.)

▶ **(6) The Base of the Skull**

This point is located at the back of the head, where the spine (atlas vertebra) and skull (occiput) meet. Here, the spinal cord meets the brain stem.

▶ **(7) The Roof of the Mouth**

This gate is located where the tongue meets the roof of the mouth on the hard palate, where the two main meridians, the governing and conception vessels, join. This gate is where the tongue touches the roof of the mouth when you say "le."

(7a) The Jaw   There are four minor gates in the jaw that are particularly useful for dealing with TMJ (temporal mandibular joint) problems, jaw tension, and the grinding of teeth. These problems are often results of high-stress conditions. Four points are important for dissolving the jaw: two are at the hinges of the jaw, located at the depression just in front of the lower edge of the ear; the two others are located inside the mouth, on its bottom, behind the front teeth. For the location of these last two gates, imagine lines descending from the inside corner of the

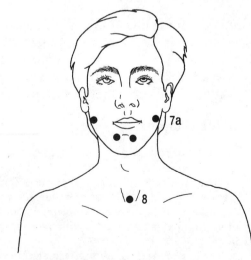

Figure 4-2 Four jaw gates and the throat notch.

eyes down to the bottom of the mouth. All four of the gates of the jaw should be dissolved simultaneously.

▶ (8) The Throat Notch

The depression just above the breast bone (the sternal notch) is the location of the last major gate of the head and neck.

▶ (9) The Seventh Cervical Vertebra

This gate is found at the big vertebra that usually sticks out at the base of the neck.

The Shoulders

▶ (1) The Shoulder Notch

This gate is found at the junction of the acromium and the clavicle; that is, at the end of the collarbone. If the arm is lifted up and to the side, it is where a depression is formed on the top of the shoulder.

▶ (2) The Armpit

This gate is in the center of the armpit, inside the body, about one-third the distance from the skin of the armpit to the shoulder notch.

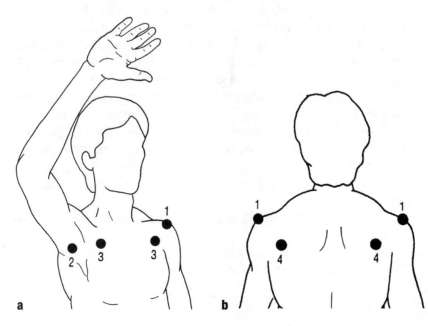

Figure 4-3 The shoulder girdle. (a) Anterior gates. (b) Posterior gates.

▶ **(3) The Shoulder's Nest**

This gate is located in the depression below the outer end of the clavicle (collarbone), lateral to the throat notch. Eventually this area will become soft and pliable, until a depression, or "nest" is formed. Most people are actually very tense and bound up here, so the depression may not be immediately noticeable. Opening this area dramatically improves flexibility in the arms. This gate is very important for women, because, together with the point in the center of the breast, it regulates the female hormonal system, especially as it affects the breast. In China, these two points are commonly used in Chi Gung treatments for breast problems, including cancer.

▶ **(4) The Center of the Shoulder Blade**

This gate is found inside the body in front of the center of the anterior (front) side of the shoulder blade (that is, the side of the shoulder blade that faces the chest).

The Arms

▶ **(1) The Elbow Joint: Back, Inside, and Sides (10 Minor Gates; 1 Major Gate)**

As the elbow, wrist, knee and ankle are the most frequently used joints in the body and must move in many directions, it is important to release the small gates surrounding each of these joints *before* releasing the main gate that is found deep in the center of each of these joints. The gates of the elbow are:

Back: the two indentations just above and the two just below the elbow tip, on either side of the tip (4 minor gates).

Inside: the two indentations just above and the two just below the crease of the elbow, on either side of the tendons (4 minor gates).

Sides: in the center of either side of the elbow (2 minor gates).

Center: directly in the middle of the elbow joint (1 major gate).

Dissolve each of the back, inside, and side gates of the elbow joint. Then dissolve the center of the joint.

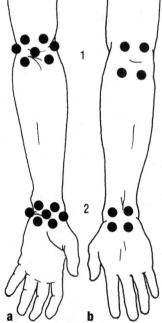

Figure 4-4 The elbows and wrists. (a) Anterior gates. (b) Posterior gates.

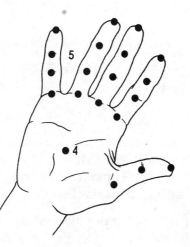

Figure 4-5 Gates of the fingers and palms.

▶ **(2) The Wrist Joint: Back, Inside, and Sides (10 Minor Gates; 1 Major Gate)**

Back: the two indentations just above and the two just below the back of the wrist joint, on either side of an imaginary line running from the middle finger to the elbow (4 minor gates).

Inside: the two indentations just above and the two just below the crease of the wrist, on either side of the tendons in the center (4 minor gates).

Sides: in the center of either side of the wrist joint (2 minor gates).

Center: in the middle of the wrist joint (1 major gate).

▶ **(3) The Carpal and Metacarpal Joints**

Dissolve all the spaces between the small bones in the palm of the hand.

▶ **(4) The Center of the Palm**

The gate in the center of the palm is commonly called the "eye of the hand." Dissolve it. Also dissolve the corresponding gate on the back of the hand. (The back-of-the-hand gate is the most critical part of the hand for those involved in any form of hands-on energetic healing.) Note: It will help to release the center of the palm if you dissolve the space between the palm and the base of the thumb.

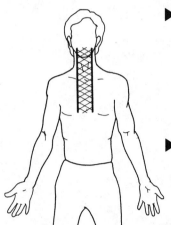

Figure 4-6 The channel from the mouth to the solar plexus.

▶ **(5) The Fingers**

In dissolving, pay particular attention to the center of the joints in the fingers. Complete the dissolving by concentrating on the exact center of the finger tips.

The Trunk

▶ **(1) From the Corners of Your Mouth, in a Channel as Wide as Your Mouth, Down the Throat and Sternum (or Breastbone) to, but Not Including, the Solar Plexus**

For the vast majority of the population, the area from where the tongue meets the roof of the mouth, down the throat to just before the solar plexus, is the most difficult for chi to pass through. This region is where the majority of people are blocked up, and it must be completely opened for any chi development practices to progress.* Special note: There are minor energy gates in the joints where the ribs attach to the sternum, in the spaces between the ribs around the sides, and in the joints where the ribs attach to the spine.

*For example, in yoga pranayama, the throat lock is used to open this area.

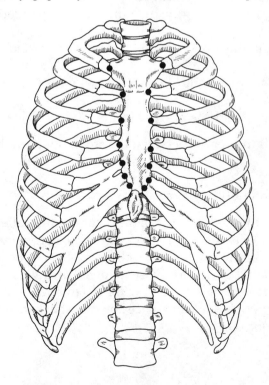

Figure 4-7 The rib cage. Minor gates at all points where ribs attach to sternum and spine.

▶ (2) The Center of the Breasts (for Women Only)

The breast gates, which have significance only for women, are extremely important for balancing the female hormonal system. These gates, along with those at the shoulder's nest, are commonly used in Chi Gung breast cancer prevention and treatment in China. These gates are located in the center of each breast, directly behind the nipple.

▶ (3) Between the Shoulder Blades

Between the shoulder blades and the spine there are a large number of minor energy gates. For athletes, dancers, and martial artists, it is extremely important to open all the gates in this area. The strength of the arms derives in large part from here, while the flexibility of the arms comes mainly from the shoulder's nest.

▶ (4) The Solar Plexus and Belly

This gate is located just below the sternum, or breastbone. It is the first soft spot you hit when you tap down the middle of breastbone.

▶ (5) The Lower *Tantien* and *Mingmen*

The lower *tantien* is located in the central core of the body, about two inches below the level of the belly button. The *mingmen* is di-

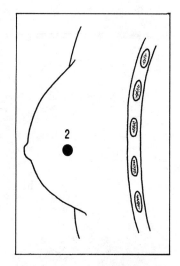

Figure 4-8 Gate at center of breast.

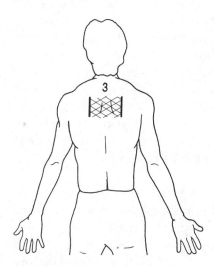

Figure 4-9 Many minor energy gates exist in the area between the shoulder blades.

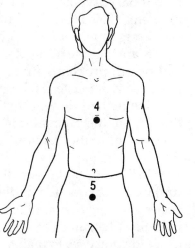

Figure 4-10 Gates at solar plexus (above) and lower tantien (below).

rectly behind the *tantien* and anterior to (just in front of) the spine.

The *tantien* is the single most important gate with regard to physical health. Located in approximately the center of the body, all energy lines related to physical health and well-being connect here.

This area is the first main focus of all Chi Gung and Taoist alchemical practices. Taoist practices all begin from the premise that physical health is the foundation upon which spiritual development is built, and it is in the lower *tantien* that all energy that affects the physical body is processed, purified, and generated. This energy can later be connected to the middle and upper tantiens for purposes of emotional and spiritual growth. Martial artists in China who did not have a deep understanding of how to use the lower *tantien* to purify their grosser emotions merely became very proficient fighting animals.

Eventually, many of the health problems caused by the premature development of the higher psychic centers can be alleviated through practices that involve the lower tantien. For this reason, most of the energy and meditation practices of Japan, China, and Korea, ranging from Zen, to Chi Gung, and to the martial arts, pay particular attention to the lower *tantien*.

Development of the energy in one *tantien* does not necessarily lead to development of the others. We have all met people who are physically healthy and emotional/psychic/spiritual wrecks. It is also common for people who are advanced on the emotional/psychic/spiritual planes to have incredible health problems. This is often because the energy of the higher centers is creating more energetic pressure than the body can handle.

Many people in the Zen community, for instance, develop bad health problems from meditation. Even the enlightened Japanese Zen master Hakuin had to go to a Taoist to repair the damage he had done to his body by prolonged sitting. Chan Buddhism, the precursor to Zen, had a very strong Chi Gung component to its practices, which was lost when it was introduced to Japan.

In Tibetan Buddhism, the initial 100,000 prostrations (nundro) have the function of developing the body before a practitioner gets into the more psychic aspects of the teachings. Yogis in India, Tibet, and China usually do some sort of physical and energetic practices to maintain the health of their bodies during their multiyear retreats, or else risk health problems.

▶ (6) The Back Muscles

Dissolve all the energy in the back muscles, especially the energy around the kidneys. Begin from the neck and shoulder area and work slowly downwards to the top of the buttocks.

▶ (7) The Spine

Beginning at the base of the skull, dissolve the entire spine, especially between the vertebrae. Pay special attention to the following locations: the place where the spine enters the skull; the big vertebrae at the base of the neck; the vertebra between the shoulder blades; the vertebra just below the shoulder blades; the vertebra level with *mingmen*; and the tailbone.

The Pelvis

▶ (1) The Pelvic Girdle

Dissolve the bones that make up the pelvic girdle; that is, the ilium, ischium, sacrum, and coccyx, especially the places where they join.

▶ (2) The Hip Socket, or Acetabulum (between the Head of the Thigh Bone and the Hip Socket).

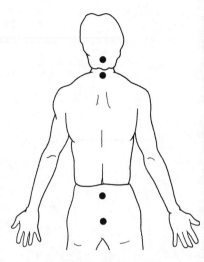

Figure 4-11 Major gates of the spine.

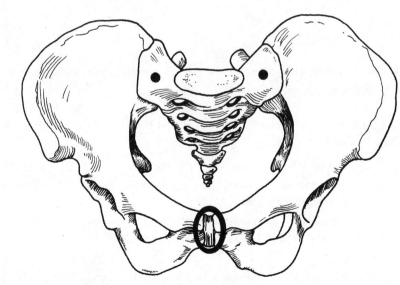

Figure 4-12 Gates of the pelvis.

▶ **(3) The Area Inside the Pelvis, Starting from the Crest of the Hip Bones All the Way through to the Inguinal Crease**

▶ **(4) The Genitals**

Men should practice the dissolving procedure up the shaft of the penis to the prostate, as well as from the testicles to the prostate. Women should dissolve the whole vaginal canal up to the cervix, but not the cervix itself. There is an energetic wall at the cervix that separates the womb from the vagina, and this *should not be dissolved.** This natural energetic seal should be broken only at childbirth. It is possible to dissolve the womb, but excessive practice can make a woman more fertile—an important issue in this era of birth control.

▶ **(5) The Anus and Rectum**

Dissolve as far up the anus as any blockage is felt, no more than a few inches deep. This is an extremely important gate, and is definitely helpful in relieving constipation, hemorrhoids, and preventing colon cancer.

▶ **(6) The Perineum**

Located between the genitals and the anus, the perineum is the point where energy from the legs and the body joins.

The Legs

The legs and buttocks support the spine, both physically and energetically.

▶ **(1) The Knee Joint: Front, Back and Sides (10 Minor Gates; 1 Major Gate)**

Front: the eyes of the knee; that is, the two indentations just above and the two just below the kneecap, on either side of the kneecap (4 minor gates).

Back: beneath the tendons on either side of the back of the knee, above and below the crease (4 minor gates).

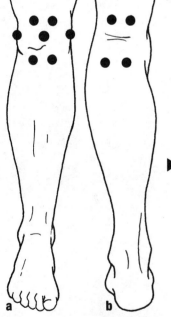

Figure 4-13 Gates of the knee. (a) Front and sides. (b) Back.

*Dissolving this area can disrupt a woman's reproductive energy and may subsequently lead to menstrual problems, PMS, vaginal infections, and the inability to conceive.

Sides: in the center of either side of the knee (2 minor gates)
Center: directly in the middle of the knee joint (1 major gate).

▶ (2) The Ankle Joint: Front, Back and Sides (8 Minor Gates; 1 Major Gate)

Front: just above and below the crease formed by pulling the foot up, on either side of the centerline of the shin bone (4 minor gates).

Back: just above the point of insertion of the achilles tendon into the heel bone, on either side (2 minor gates).

Sides: in the center of the ankle bone on either side (2 minor gates).

Center: directly in the middle of the ankle joint (1 major gate).

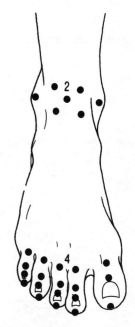

Figure 4-14 Gates of the ankles and toes.

▶ (3) The Tarsals and Metatarsals

Dissolve all the spaces between the small bones of the foot.

▶ (4) The Toes

Dissolve all the toe joints, up to and especially including the tips of the toes.

▶ (5) The Heel

About one inch from the very back of the foot, on the center line of the foot.

▶ (6) The Arch

In the center of the arch, on the midline of the foot (inside the foot).

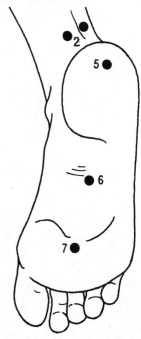

▶ (7) The Bubbling Well

About one-third the distance from the base of the toes to the heel, on the bottom of the foot. This gate is in the depression formed when you point your toes. It is on the midline of the foot.

Figure 4-15 Major gates of the bottom of the foot and the back of the ankle.

Below the Feet and Above the Head

Your energetic body extends below your feet and above your head. The size of your energetic body, unlike your physical body, grows and shrinks with time. It is in constant flux. Over time, and with practice, your energy body will grow in size and strength, but it will still fluctuate.

Feel below your body until you can't feel anymore, until you find where your energy body has reached its natural end. Dissolve the energy from the bottom of your feet downward until the energy ends. No matter in what environment you find yourself, always dissolve to the ends of your energy body.

Your energy body also ends above your head. (Some of the Yoga traditions refer to the eighth and ninth chakras, located above the head.)

Feel above your head until the sense of energy ends. This is where you will now begin all dissolving practices. One complete standing exercise will constitute dissolving the energy from above the head, through the body, and culminate with all of the energy dissolving into the energy point below your feet; that is, your root. After standing, open your eyes slowly, making sure that they open at your internal speed.

Opening the Gates: A Lesson Plan

Each lesson should be practiced for at least three days, or as long as you need to stabilize the gate or gates referred to in the lesson Moving too fast creates strain and scatters energy, resulting in little benefit.

First, lightly dissolve all gates you have previously opened, and then spend the remaining 80% of your practice time on opening the new energy gates below. It is important to dissolve all the blocked energy above the new gates; this includes not just the energy that is blocked at the major gates, but energy blocked anywhere else as well. For example, when moving from the crown to the third eye be sure to dissolve the forehead, and when moving from the hips to the knees be sure to dissolve the thighs.

If you feel that too much material is contained in one lesson, just divide it up. Go at your own pace—there is no pressure to complete this process in any specific amount of time. Generally speaking, allow at least four to twelve weeks to work your way down through all the gates to your feet.

At the end of any practice session, gently dissolve through the rest of the body to the floor.

Suggested lessons for dissolving (each number consists of one lesson) are below.

1. *Bai hwei*, or the crown of the head
2. The third eye, the eyes, the center of the ears, and the temple. Also, the four jaw points (see p. 64).
3. Where the tongue touches the roof of the mouth and the throat notch
4. The base of the skull and in between each of the cervical (neck) vertebrae down to the seventh cervical vertebra at the base of the neck
5. From where the tongue touches the roof of your mouth to the end of the breastbone, on a line about the width of your mouth
6. The four points of the shoulder
7. The elbows
8. The wrists
9. The hands (all the points)
10. The joints where the ribs connect to the sternum, the spaces between the ribs, the joints where the ribs connect to the spine, the area between the shoulder blades and the spine. For women only: the gates of the breasts (directly behind the nipples)
11. The solar plexus
12. The whole of the belly, starting from the front and dissolving through the internal organs back to the spine
13. The *tantien* and the *mingmen*
14. All the points along the spine, from the occiput to the tailbone, paying special attention to the occiput, the seventh cervical vertebra; the vertebra in the center of shoulder blades, the one at the base of the shoulder blades, *mingmen* and the tailbone.
15. The hip sockets, the pelvic bones, and the kwa (that is, the area inside the front crest of the hip bones)
16. The anus
17. The genitals
18. The perineum
19. The knees

20. The ankles
21. The feet
22. Below the floor
23. Above the head

After completing this sequence, begin all further standing meditation from above the head, and dissolve down the body one level at a time. Imagine the body to be full of water, with the water being slowly let out from the bottom of your feet. As the water level drops, dissolve everything at the new level—front, back, and side.

When dissolving the crown of the head, then, you want to dissolve everything else at the same level; that is, the entire top of your head. As you work towards the next gate, the third eye, dissolve down the head so that all sides of the head at the same level are dissolved simultaneously. At the solar plexus, then, you would also be working on the lower ribs, those vertebrae at the level of the lower ribs, and the elbows (approximately).

Guidelines for the Practice of Standing Chi Gung

Don't Overstrain Your Energy System

Release as much as possible of the blocked ("stuck") energy above the gate you are working on and drop what remains into the next lower gate. Continue on down through successive lower gates to below the floor. Spend three or four days until the mind has become reasonably stable there. Work slowly on each gate (or series of gates), releasing enough energy above each new gate so that energy can be released from the gate itself without over-straining the system. If you go too fast, it creates strain—energy is scattered and little progress is made.

Dissolve from the Skin Inward

In general, begin on the outer surface of the body, and over the next months begin to go deeper and deeper, until you gain a direct experience of the bones. Also, remember that during the first month or two, you should not go more than one-half inch into the brain, though later it is permissible to extend the dissolving process through the entire brain. Just be sure *not* to do anything specific with the chi of gates you encounter inside the brain, such as making connections or geometric patterns.

Allow Six Months to Stabilize the Tantien and Mingmen

Moving down through the gates of the body to the *tantien* will usually take at least a month, it will probably be another month before the *tantien* stabilizes (fixes in location), and it will take anywhere from three to six months before you will be able to extend your mind from the *tantien* (in the center) to the *mingmen* (on the spine). It will also take three to six months to begin to store energy in the *tantien*. (This process can be accelerated when studying with a master, and may take longer on your own.)

The Legs Are More Difficult than the Arms

In general, especially for Westerners, the legs will be more difficult to open than the arms, as we in the West tend to focus on our heads and upper bodies. Also, we do not tend to sit or squat on the floor. Because Westerners do not tend to direct chi into their legs, the legs become insensitive to energy.

Stand a Minimum of Five Minutes to Get Benefits

As a general rule, a minimum of five minutes standing is necessary for any noticeable results. This presupposes that a person is able to drop into a state of complete relaxation in thirty or forty seconds, and after a few months of practice this is a highly realistic goal. In the beginning, however, it may take five minutes to attain a reasonable state of relaxation. If this is so, those five minutes must be added to the practice time; in other words, ten minutes would be necessary for any benefit to accrue. On a super-stressed day, you might require fifteen minutes just to relax enough to begin the standing practice.

　　The longest I have seen people do standing and still gain benefit from it is about six hours at a time.* For the average per-

---

*For about a year and a half while I was at Sophia University, I would quite commonly practice for about six hours at a time. However, it must be borne in mind that I was about 20 years old and had only school work to do, so I had lots of free time and little stress in my life.

son, standing beyond one hour at a time usually is impractical, and therefore one hour can be considered a maximum practice time. To reach this amount, gradually increase the length of practice by two or three minutes every day, or even every week or month.

Now, obviously, if you can only practice five, ten, or fifteen minutes a day during the week and then do an hour or two on a weekend, your muscles may become sore. A half an hour might be called for, but not much more until you have built up to it. Never strain yourself internally. Slow, steady, even, and with moderation should be the key guidelines for the average person, who wants to maintain or improve health, flexibility, and well-being. Of course, these principles also apply to martial artists and athletes, but what is moderate for them, the average person would no doubt find somewhat excessive.

Standing for People Involved in Movement Arts

Since the movement arts require superior flexibility and body control, people involved in these arts should do a minimum of twenty minutes standing at a time, up to a maximum of two hours, depending upon how strong they want their energy to be and how deeply they desire total command and knowledge of their physical being. Practicing in this range will take one beyond mere physical maintenance to a level of superior physical ability. For those under 25, the amount of practice time could quite possibly be increased, whereas those over 50 might want to start with a little less.

Always bear in mind never to overstrain, as this can create an internal resistance to practicing. If the body or mind is pushed too far in one direction it will naturally snap back in the other direction. Consistent practice will get you much further than periodic blasts, which often cause your practice time to dramatically diminish. A two-and-a-half hour practice marathon could be so internally exhausting that the internal resistance to further exhaustion would prevent practice for the next week or so.

Standing for Martial Artists and Healers

The martial artist should be aware that the standing posture has been used in China for thousands of years to develop internal power. At more advanced stages, there are many hand postures that open up every energy line in the body and allow the manifestation of internal power from any part of the body at will. As part of traditional Chinese healing and body work (Twei Na) there are approximately 200 different hand postures, each with different mind components, which are capable of healing the damage caused by illness and injury. Each of these postures deals with a specific way in which energy is not moving through the system. With practice, it is possible to make energy move through any blockage in the system, whether in internal organs, nerve tissue, soft tissue, or the spine.

When I was younger I practiced six hours at a stretch in order to increase my internal power. At that time I was actively involved in fighting competitions where it was easy to get severely hurt, and this significantly increased my motivation to learn. If I did not practice hard enough, I was realistically looking at an opponent putting me in the hospital. Now, most people do not have this strong a motivation, and the majority of people practicing the internal martial arts are not in their late teens and early twenties. Therefore, I would say that between one and three hours a day is the maximum that the average dedicated martial artist or healer should be practicing.

Do Not Stand Too Long

It is important to realize that there is a point of diminishing returns, beyond which the extra practice doesn't really result in enough benefit to be worth it. Again, beware of the internal exhaustion factor: If you get too internally exhausted, you will not be able to practice for days. So find where this maximum benefit point is for you and don't go beyond it. It is normal to learn through the school of hard knocks where your limits are. Internal exhaustion is infinitely more tiring than exhaustion attained through external exercise, including marathon running—it is like nervous exhaustion combined with physical exhaustion.

Dissolve Your Energy Blocks at Progressively Deeper Levels

The average practice period consists of a period of settling in, followed by a period where everything feels wrong and you begin concentrating on the weakest (most obviously bound-up) link in your chain. Then, after feeling like you've unknotted that block, a tremendous sense of liberated energy is felt moving within. The point at which this liberated energy begins to weaken is when most people call it a day. However, after much practice (months to years), it is possible to find a second weak link, dissolve it, and get a new burst of energy. Only the most experienced practitioners can go through this cycle three or four times, and these people are rare.

Again, the keys are consistency and not overdoing it. If these are adhered to, standing can give a martial artist or athlete an easy, relaxed, and effortless power that cannot be gained through any amount of physical training or weight lifting.

Cloud Hands:
Rooting the Lower Body

Cloud Hands Is the Most Complete
Chi Gung Movement

Cloud Hands contains all of the same essential energy elements that make Tai Chi Chuan the highly effective system of healing that it is. If you could only practice one single move for health, Cloud Hands would be it. It involves both the arms and the legs in forward, backward, up, and down motions, and includes all of Tai Chi's basic twisting, turning, bending, and stretching motions. Although there is no shifting of the weight forward and back, the weight does shift completely from one side to the other, and thus Cloud Hands contains the basic process of moving from empty to full. The principles learned in Cloud Hands also apply to Hsing I, Ba Gua, and the vast majority of Chi Gung and Nei Gung exercises.

In the different styles of Tai Chi Chuan, Cloud Hands is performed in many different ways. The Cloud Hands described here is fairly simple, and derives from an original Taoist practice that contains all the internal principles (without necessarily the specific form) of the Yang, Wu, Chen, and combination Tai Chi/Hsing I/Ba Gua styles.

Beginning with the feet and working up to the hands, this exercise will be taught in a number of stages, each of which incorporates essential internal principles.

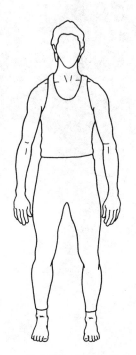

Figure 5-1 Standing posture.

Instructions for the Cloud Hands Movement

▶ **(1) Gently Open Your Eyes**

When standing (Fig. 5-1) with your eyes closed, dissolving internal blockages, it is quite natural to go into a light trance. In time, this light trance state will pass, as internal clarity becomes stronger. In the beginning, however, it is normal to slow down and become extremely relaxed.

After standing, slowly open your eyes, making sure that they open at your internal speed. Your entrance into the world of sight should be a gradual and comfortable one. In order to do this, open your eyes at the same internal speed that you have previously been experiencing your insides. The object is to have a smooth transition from internal awareness to external awareness, avoiding a shock similar to that which individuals would experience if they were to come from a dark cave and suddenly open their eyes to bright sunlight, or cold water were thrown on them while in a deep sleep. Maintaining the relaxation and internal sense of openness experienced in standing as you transit into moving allows you to carry over this relaxation into movement. Thus, the movement can increase relaxation and develop even more energy.

▶ **(2) Begin Cloud Hands**

Place your feet parallel to each other, shoulder-width apart. With your eyes open and your feet parallel, shift all your weight (100% of it) to your weaker leg, let's say the left. Keeping the weight there, extend your right leg to the side a few inches, maintaining both feet parallel (Fig. 5-2a). Keep the weight on the weighted foot (in this case, the left) evenly distributed, so that no one part has any more or less weight than any other. Then extend your energy and your weight through your feet to the point below the floor where your energy body ends; that is, your root. If you are able to extend your energy below the floor, the energy of the earth will naturally connect with your body's energy. You will then be able to draw energy into your body from the earth just as a tree does, as well as circulate chi from the left to the right side of your body and from right to left when you shift weight to the opposite foot.

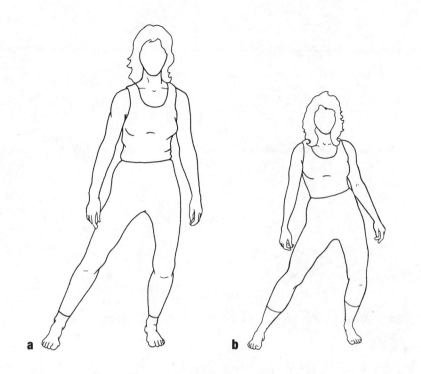

Figure 5-2 Weight 100% on left leg. (a) Correct: hips level. (b) Incorrect: hips tilted.

▶ (3) Tuck the Pelvis and Slowly Shift Weight

Next, check that your pelvis is tucked under and that your lower back is straight. Begin to shift your weight 100% from left leg to right leg, and right leg to left leg back and forth, a number of times. (Most people will find that their leg muscles will ache after a while; this is only natural.) The shifting must be slow and steady, and as far as possible free of any jerks or spasms, and speed should remain constant throughout the shift. Check that your hips remain even, parallel to the floor, and are not shifting up or down with the movement.

▶ (4) The 70% Rule (as Applied to Leg Width)

The first question that often comes to mind has to do with how far apart to put the legs. And now we come to a fundamental principle concerning how these, and all Taoist exercises, are done: the 70% Rule. In any Tai Chi or Chi Gung Core Exercise, first estimate what 100% of your physical capacity is in terms of

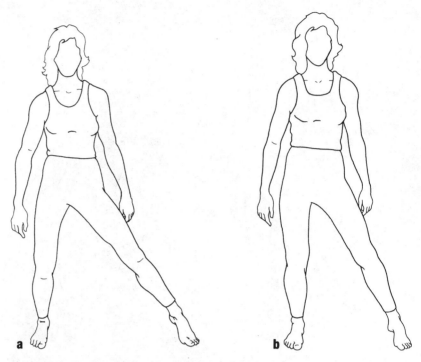

Figure 5-3 The 70% rule. (a) Leg width is at 100% of capacity. (b) Leg width brought back to 70% of capacity.

range of movement or time of practice; that is, how far your body can actually stretch and how much your body can endure before it collapses. Once you determine this, you then only move or practice to 70% of your capacity (Fig. 5-3b). This percentage is not rigid, and the appropriate amount could be anywhere from 60 to 80%, depending on your condition.

If people were totally sensitive and aware of all their internal limitations, there probably wouldn't be much of a need to mention this rule. The principle upon which the 70% rule is based is that development must begin by considering your weakest link. Do not seek maximum performance, as that quest may both damage the weak link and cause the whole system to contract and tense up.

The "Give 100%" Attitude Is Dangerous

Commonly, when people try to give 100%, they inadvertently go to 110 or 120% of their body's maximum capacity, which results in injury, sometimes slight and sometimes severe. We've all heard of the beginning runner who goes out on his first day knowing he needs to warm up. He stretches his legs, starts running, reaches 100% of his capacity without knowing it, and when he decides to go a little further ("more is better") he pulls his hamstring. Three weeks later he tries again, maybe a little wiser, but most likely not.

Another factor is at work here. At 70% of your perceived performance level, you can throw 100% of your energy and effort into developing what you are practicing. Yet as you approach 100% of capacity, the body will subconsciously react with fear to potential damage. This fear is a necessary and natural survival mechanism, and even without your awareness, your body and mind will tense up in response to it. Since two of the fundamental purposes of the core exercises are to develop deep relaxation and reduce stress in the body, this 100% attitude is counterproductive.

Many athletes will overtrain to win, resulting in permanent damage to their bodies. This is opposite to the principles of the Core Exercises, which aim to make your body and mind work in a more relaxed, efficient, and healthy manner for the rest of your life. The more you practice them, the more energy you have—so long as you keep within the 70% rule. The 70% rule prevents people from becoming heroes at the expense of their bodies.

Moderation Protects Old Injuries

Many people with weak knees, bad ankles, or old injuries (which they may even be unaware of), will find that keeping to this principle of moderation will save a lot of physical pain and bodily damage, whether doing Chi Gung or any other type of exercise. The majority of Americans do not have a regular exercise regimen, and therefore try to do everything in the first week, or even the first day. Now the one thing all athletes know is that you often do not know what injuries have occurred until the next day. The purpose of the 70% rule is to prevent injuries before they occur.

It has been my experience, having taught thousands of people, that a whole lot of people ignore these safety warnings even after several injuries! It is my hope that you will re-read the 70%

rule at least three or four times, and take note of when your body speaks to you. It would prefer that you didn't damage it.

How to Shift Weight from Side to Side

You will find it very helpful to practice the weight-shifting motion with one or two other people. In this particular exercise, have one person check that your lower back is straight, and the other person watch that your hips move from side to side without going up and down. Also, have your partner make sure that your body does not rise and fall as you shift your weight from side to side. Make sure that both feet are completely flat on the floor (except the arch, of course), and that all parts of the sole of the foot touch the floor equally. The weight should not ride on the inner or outer edge of the foot, forward on the ball of the foot, or backward on the heel.

Mechanics of the Joints

Now let's consider the alignment of the joints of the leg. We will start with the ankles, but the principles stated here will apply to all joints of the body.

The fundamental structure of a human joint is a ball and socket. A ball and socket is like a mortar and pestle and, as with a mortar and pestle, the object is to squeeze or grind up the contents contained and not the container.

Human joints, likewise, are not designed to have the ball grind on the socket. In the joints, there is a substance called synovial fluid, which is capable of tremendous compression. This fluid acts as a buffer between the ball and the socket, and compresses and expands in proportion to the amount of pressure put on it.

One basic function of muscles is to keep the alignment of the bones in a joint stable, so that the joint's natural hydraulic abilities can manifest. If the ball and the socket fit evenly into each other, the joint will receive a bare minimum of shock no matter what action is performed.

Human beings were meant to be able to walk on their legs for 70 to 80 years. They were meant to be able to move things with their arms millions of times in a lifetime. Your joints will not wear out if the internal pressure of the synovial fluid is kept constant and if the ball and socket joints remain aligned. However, if the proper alignment is lost, the ball can slowly damage the socket, or vice versa. The supporting ligaments, muscles, and tendons can then become overstretched or damaged, resulting in further misalignment. This vicious cycle causes the joints to weaken and lose their natural capacity to function. Thus, a person can eventually become arthritic or too weak to do even the simplest tasks.

The Negative Effects of Joint Problems on the Whole Body

According to Chinese medical thinking and the science of chi development, when problems begin in a joint, energy begins to stagnate there, so that it cannot circulate to the rest of the system. This situation causes a number of extremely negative effects. First of all, local blood circulation is decreased, which then decreases the circulation throughout the body. Secondly, as the chi or energy of the body stagnates in the joint, the internal organs do not receive as much energy as they need. Thirdly, though the joint has plenty of coagulated energy, it is still starved of good energy, and it thus begins to pull energy from healthy tissues of the body, thereby weakening those tissues.

The sequence of the weakening of the tissues is: The stagnated joints pull energy from other joints, then from the organs, then from the spine, and then from the brain. So one of the first goals of the Chi Gung Core Exercises is to release bound-up joints; then energy can flow smoothly through the system.

Proper Alignment of the Knee Joint

Both in standing and in the initial movement from side to side, make sure that all parts of your foot (aside from the arch) are touching the floor equally. When one part of your foot raises or collapses, this is a clear sign that the ankle joint is not aligned. Also check to make sure that your knee joint is aligned with your ankle (Figs. 5-4a, b). Realize that it is the shin that connects your knee to your ankle. In order for this connection to be solid, the

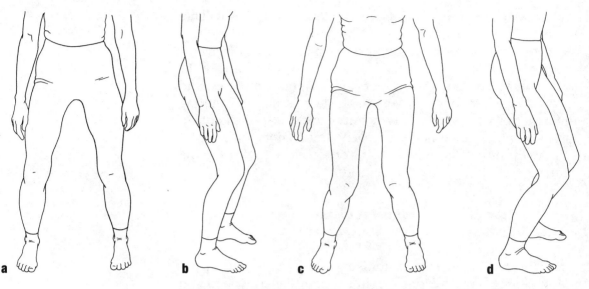

Figure 5-4 Knee alignment. (a) and (b) Correct: center of knee above center of foot. (c) Incorrect: knees collapsed inward. (d) Incorrect: knees collapsed forward.

line from the knee to the ankle in the weight bearing leg must be stable and at a 90° angle to the floor. When viewed from the front, a vertical line dropped from the center of your patella (kneecap) directly downwards should go through the center of your ankle.

▶ The Knee Is a Weight-Transference Joint, Not a Weight-Bearing Joint

An extension of the above consideration is that if someone were to push downwards on the crest of the hip from the side of your body, the alignment of the body should be such that the pressure goes directly into the center of the arch of the foot. No pressure should be felt in the knee joints—*the knee is a weight-transference joint, not a weight-bearing joint.*

When the knee joint is properly aligned, there is a feeling of tremendous springiness, not unlike that felt when using a bicycle pump or pushing on the brakes of a car. This springiness does not require any physical exertion, as the alignment itself will create the springiness.

▶ **How to Test the Knee Joint**

There is a simple exercise to help you acquire this sensation. Have a partner gently push down on your thigh and into your knee as you shift from side to side. This will lead to the discovery that only one or two of the many possible positions of your knee and ankle will be comfortable and stable. Don't push with so great a force as to risk injury; the object is purely to find where the knee and ankle alignment is stable and springy.

Practice going from side to side with a partner until both of you are able to recognize the proper joint alignment. Remember to find this alignment whenever you practice internal energy exercises of any nature, or, for that matter, any normal athletic activities. This particular technique generally makes a huge difference to skiers and participants in other sports where tremendous pressure is exerted on the knees and ankles.

▶ **Open the Back of the Knee Joint**

Other knee problems suffered by all sorts of athletes, as well as Chi Gung and Tai Chi practitioners, are caused by not properly opening up the back of the knee. Most people bend their knees in such a way as to put all the stress into the front of the knee, which structurally is very weak. The back of the knee closes while the front of the knee opens, creating a very small "V" shape. The pressure on the front of the knee slowly pulls out some of the soft tissue (ligaments, muscles, tendons) and creates knee problems. This can be thought of as a self-inflicted knee lock, functioning just like a wrist lock or elbow twist.

▶ **Exercise to Align the Knee and Ankle Joints**

Here is another helpful exercise to align the joints of the knees and ankles. Working with a partner, lie on the floor and lift one leg up to chest height. Your partner grabs the heel and ball of your foot and pushes forward (not hard). You must discover the alignment of the knee, ankle, and kwa (hip fold, pronounced "kwah"), which uses the natural pressure of the synovial fluid, to push back with the bare minimum of effort (Fig. 5-5a). Rely on the springiness of the joint, rather than the muscles. If the joint is not aligned properly, the experience will be one of muscle strain and discomfort, and if the joint is really out of line, there will also be pain. If, however, the foot, ankle, knee, and kwa are

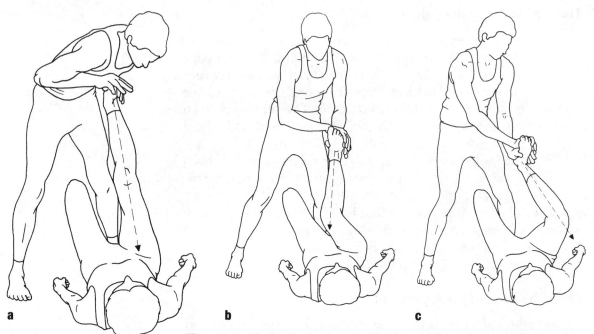

Figure 5-5 Aligning the knee and ankle joints. (a) Correct: hip, knee, and ankle joints in a line. (b) Incorrect: knee collapsed inward. (c) Incorrect: knee turned outward.

properly aligned, you will be able effortlessly to push several people away from you with your leg.

If you have had any back, knee, or ankle injuries, be very gentle throughout these exercises, as you are only trying to find the difference between the ease and comfort of a properly aligned joint and the strain and discomfort of an improperly aligned one. Human beings were designed to be able to walk for many miles without great effort. With these exercises, you are simply becoming conscious of the mechanisms that allow the body to function optimally.

Opening and Closing the Kwa

The area of the body that the Chinese call the kwa extends from the inguinal ligament through the inside of the pelvis to the top (crest) of the hip bones. Included within the kwa are (1) the left and right channels of energy; (2) the pelvis, including the hip joint; (3) the sacrum and first few lumbar vertebrae; (4) the il-

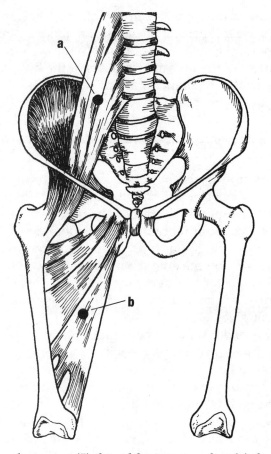

Figure 5-6 Deep muscles of the kwa. (a) iliopsoas group. (b) adductor group.

iopsoas muscle group; (5) the adductor muscles; (6) the pelvic diaphragms (the health of which is essential to sexual vitality); (7) the lower intestine; and (8) the rectum.

The muscles of the kwa (Fig. 5-6) connect the legs to the spine: the iliopsoas connects the lumbar vertebrae to the pelvis and femur (thigh bone), and the adductors connect the pelvis to the femur. The springiness of the spine and legs is partially determined by the elasticity of the iliopsoas muscles. Many lower back problems are caused by stiffness, spasm, or trauma in the iliopsoas muscles.

At the inguinal groove, the largest collection of lymph nodes in the body can be found. Lymph is a critical component of the body's immune response system. Unlike blood, which is moved by the heart and vascular system, lymph is basically moved by muscular contractions. Nature is very wise—every time we walk or move our legs and arms, large lymph collectors (at the inguinal groove, or in the armpits, for example) are activated, thus moving our lymph. Chinese Nei Gung exercises simply increase this natural phenomenon, thereby strengthening a very important component of the immune system. Increasing the movement of the internal elements of the kwa is one of the most significant and unique contributions to health of all the chi-enhancing body practices.

The Kwa Squat Exercise

Begin by assuming the basic standing posture described in Chapter 3. Make sure you maintain all the proper structural alignments. Be especially careful to align the knees and ankles, with all points of your foot touching the floor evenly. Check the alignment by sinking your hips to see if you can feel your hips directly pressing on the arch of your foot. All weight and pressure should transfer through your knee and ankle joints to the foot. Bounce lightly, using your hips so that you can feel the spring in your legs.

For this exercise, the knees must remain fixed in space, moving neither forward nor backward, both going up and down. This can be checked in several ways: have a partner position his or her arm in front of your knee caps, or use a chair or a piece of string. It is important that, whatever feedback method you choose, you do not use a rigid or immovable object like a wall or a heavy piece of furniture. You want to find out if your knee caps are moving in space, but you don't want to put pressure on them.

Squat down by squeezing your kwa closed, and stand up by expanding or pushing your kwa upward. Under no circumstances should you use your knees to power your squat. There must be a direct line of pressure from your kwa to the arch of your foot, with no weight-bearing pressure exerted on the knees. Squat only as low as you can go without the knees moving forward. If the knees move forward, weight can go into the knee joint, possibly causing injury. The spine must remain straight (without the back muscles being tensed). The spine may incline forward on an angle (as minimal as your body will allow), but your back must not arch. Be sure to keep the perineum open and relax your legs. The squeezing of the kwa is similar to (but not exactly the same as) the way one squeezes to prevent one's bowel movements.

You may be able to squat only an inch or two in the beginning. People with weak, stiff, or traumatized psoas muscles will be surprised by how little they can squat. This is nothing to worry about. In time, your body will regain the same flexibility seen in a child's ability to squat.

Remember: squat only as low as you can go without the knees moving forward. Squatting to where the buttocks are even with the knees is about the lowest one should want to go. A good practice is to use this kwa squat to pick things up off the floor or from low shelves, or for lifting or putting down heavy objects.

Developing the flexibility of the kwa is essential for Nei Gung, Taoist energy and meditation practices, and the internal martial arts, including Tai Chi Chuan. This simple squatting exercise is an excellent way to begin stretching the muscles of the kwa and start developing that elastic quality.

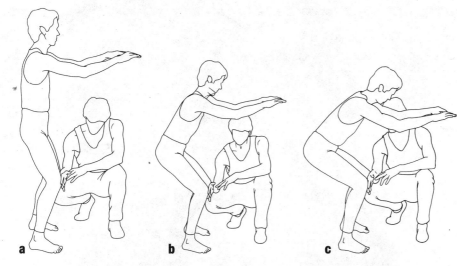 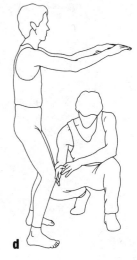

Figure 5-7 Kwa Squat. (a) Stand as in the posture from Chapter Three, with both feet parallel. Partner places forearm and hand on both knees. Partner does not move his forearm during the whole exercise. Your knees must continue to touch his forearm during the whole exercise, both going up and down.
(b) Squeeze Kwa closed and squat. Spine must remain straight, not arched, and arms may be held straight in front of body, with body inclined forward to aid balance. (c) Maintain the conditions of (a) and (b), squeeze Kwa, and squat lower. If you are stiff or have an injured back, it may take months to squat this low.
(d) Maintain the conditions of 5-7(a), open Kwa, and stand up. Make sure your knees do not move.

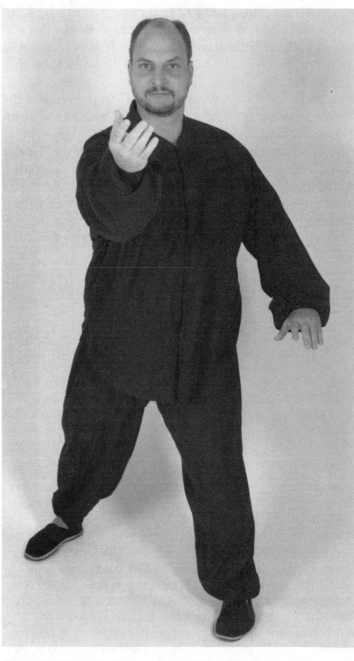

The author shows the final extension of Cloud Hands.

CHAPTER 6

Cloud Hands:
Spiraling the Upper Body

The Spine Connects the Arms and the Legs

A basic function of the Cloud Hands exercise is to connect the energy of your whole body to your spine, which results in the nerves of the spine integrating with the entire body without breaks or dysfunction. This is achieved in three steps.

First, the legs are joined energetically to the pelvis and then to the spine. (You learned how to accomplish this is Chapter 5.) The energy that supports your spine comes from the earth through your legs.

Second, the arms are joined energetically to the spine—you will learn how this is accomplished in this chapter.

Third, the energies from the arms and legs are integrated with each other, through the spine. At this stage, it is very important that the Heaven and Earth energy connection—from above the head to below the feet—be kept strong during the movements of Cloud Hands.

The arms and the legs are essentially the same from the viewpoint of the spine. The hip/shoulder, elbow/knee, and hand/foot have approximately the same vertical and horizontal movements. The coordination between the hands and legs is what allows multidirectional flexibility. Your legs are connected to the earth, and your arms to heaven.

First Exercise: Connecting the Arms to the Spine

This technique involves sinking the shoulders and dropping the elbows.

Instructions for the First Exercise

▶ **(1) Raise Arms**

To begin, raise your arms forward to shoulder height, with the wrists and elbows bent and the hands and fingers parallel to the floor, palms down (Fig. 6-1a). The forearms and the upper arms should be parallel to each other; do not let them make a "V" shape, either out or in. Make sure the tips of your elbows point

Figure 6-1 Raising arms to shoulder height. (a) Correct: elbows bent. (b) Incorrect: arms straight. (c) Incorrect: left arm properly aligned with side channel, but right arm turned out. (d) Incorrect: left arm slightly turned out, right arm extremely turned out.

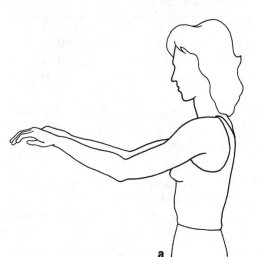

a

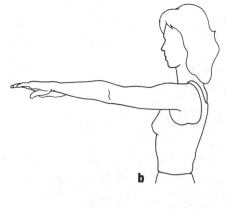

b

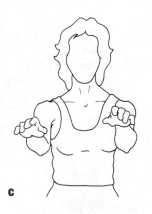

c

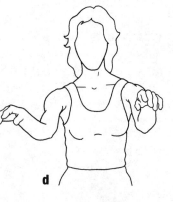

d

directly to the ground, so that the upper arms, elbows, and fore-arms are parallel to each other. The object is to have each arm from shoulder to fingers remain on the right and left energy channels of the body (which extend from the shoulder nests down to the kwa on each side).

▶ (2) Open the Shoulder Blades

Next, relax your shoulders, letting them drop down, while at the same time rounding the shoulder blades and the back as far as possible. When this movement is done properly, the shoulder blades will seem to disappear.

▶ (3) Sink Elbows

Let your elbows drop slightly as if weights were attached to them, pulling them down (Fig. 6-2a). In order to do this, the area the Chinese call the "shoulder's nest" must be opened, creating a hollow between the inner edge of the shoulder and the ribs. This area, in time, becomes extremely soft and very flexible. When this hollow is produced in the shoulder's nest, the shoulders sink and the elbows drop easily and comfortably, without conscious thought.

These steps are all intimately connected, and function primarily to connect the arms energetically to the spine, much like branches grow out of a tree trunk and are not separate from the tree. Most people lack a strong sense of energetic connection between the spine and the arms. Without such connection, the chi from the spine will have difficulty flowing past the shoulders;

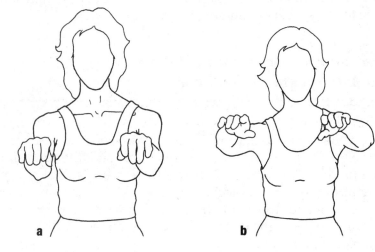

a   b

Figure 6-2 Sinking the elbows. (a) Correct: elbow tips point down. (b) Incorrect: elbows turned out.

thus, true energy work will be prevented and the exercise will be limited to muscular activity only.

▶ **(4) Practice the First Exercise, Moving with Arms Raised**

Close your eyes and shift weight from side to side, with your arms in the position indicated in Step 1. You will find that, after a few minutes, your arms probably will have spread out into a "V" shape. Practice this exercise from a few days up to two weeks, until your arms move only with your body and spine, and not independently, remaining parallel. Without practicing this exercise, it is very difficult to get your arms to move in accord with your spine. The exercise stabilizes the flow of chi from the spine to the arms.

▶ **Two-Person Feedback Exercise**

During the practice of this exercise (and some of the others) it is useful to have a partner check to see if you are actually doing what you think you are doing. It is more useful to ask a partner than to look in a mirror. When someone else places you in the correct position, it is possible to compare the way it feels to do an exercise correctly with the way it feels when you think you are doing it correctly. One problem with looking in a mirror is that you are not only doing the exercise, you also are watching, so already there is some dissociation from the feeling in your arms. Second, it is very common to look in a mirror and see only what you want to see. Also, you usually won't have a mirror to practice with, and it is much more important to gain an inner sense of the correct movements and postures. So, if possible, find someone to work with as you practice these exercises.

Second Exercise: Move the Elbow Joints to Activate the Spinal Pump

The objective of this next exercise is to link the opening and closing of the elbows to the opening and closing of all the tissue from the elbow to the spine (i.e., the upper arm, shoulder, and shoulder blade). The exercise activates the cerebro-spinal pump in the upper spine and neck, which works in association with increasing and decreasing the space between the vertebrae (as the arms extend, the distance increases, and as they contract, it decreases).

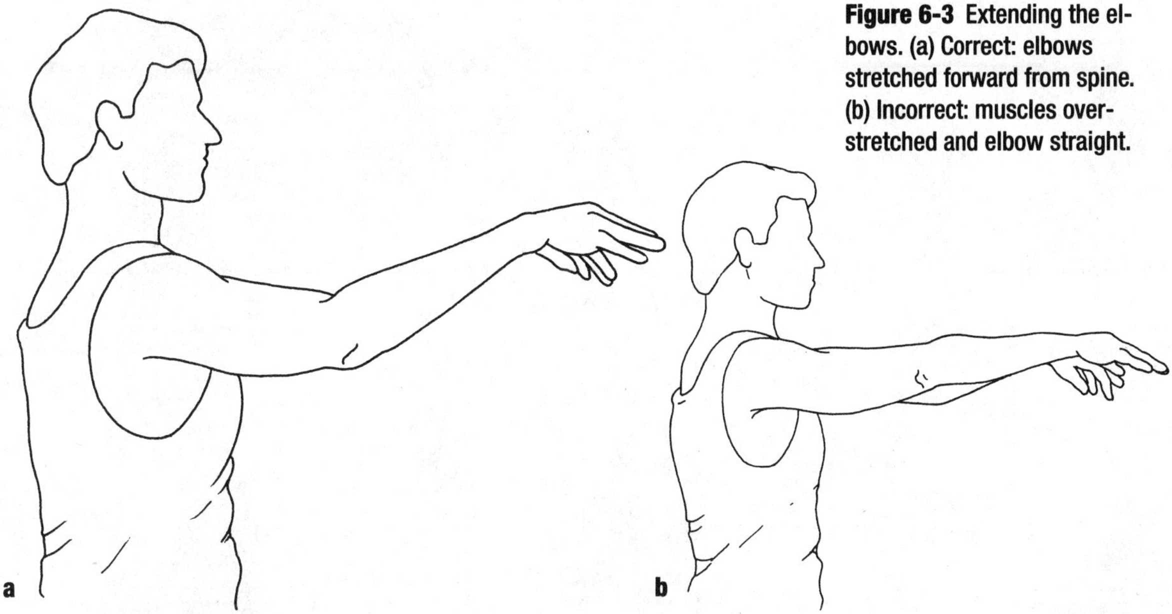

Figure 6-3 Extending the elbows. (a) Correct: elbows stretched forward from spine. (b) Incorrect: muscles overstretched and elbow straight.

a   b

▶ (1) Extend the Elbows

The procedure is as follows: while keeping the shoulders down, extend the elbows as far forward as possible, so that all the tissue from the spine through the shoulder blades to the shoulder notch is as stretched and open as possible (Fig. 6-3a). This extension must not decrease at any point in this exercise—never allow any slack from the elbow to the spine. Simply, your elbow can stay put or extend further, but must not contract. The muscles must not become tense or overstretched. Like a rubber band, the muscles from your spine to your fingers must be as extended as far as possible so there is no slack in them. Yet, also like a rubber band, not so taut that the rubber becomes ready to snap (pull the muscle). Remember the 70% rule.

▶ (2) Open and Close the Elbow Joints to Activate the Spinal Pump

Now bend and straighten the arms to activate the spinal pump and consequent stretching of the vertebrae (remember to only extend and bend to 70% of your limit). When you can feel the action of this exercise from the mid-thoracic vertebrae (between the shoulder blades) to the top of the neck, you have learned

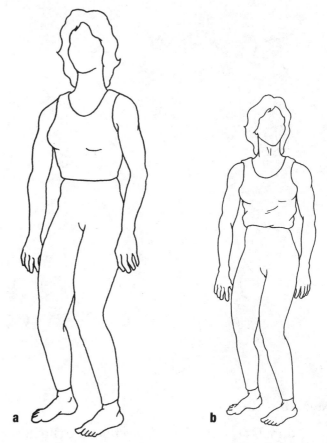

Figure 6-4 Turning the body. (a) Correct: nose, solar plexus, and groin in one line. (b) Incorrect: centerline broken.

a

b

well. This exercise is extremely difficult to learn without the help of a qualified teacher, largely because you have to feel what is going on inside your body on a very subtle level, and usually the instructor has to manipulate the student's arms before they get the exact feeling. While the internal action is extremely powerful, it is almost invisible from the outside, except to the highly trained observer.

Third Exercise: Open the Hip Joint to Turn the Spine

▶ (1) Coordinate Upper and Lower Body Turning

Now we are ready for turning movements, which means it is time to find the centerline of the body. Figure 6-4a shows proper alignment of the body while turning. Note how the centerline is maintained. Figure 6-4b shows how most people turn, breaking the centerline and thereby disengaging the upper body from the lower.

With the hands equidistant from the centerline of the body, begin to turn from side to side, remembering all the previously discussed material; that is, lower back straight, hip-knee-ankle connected, back raised, chest rounded, shoulders sunk, elbows dropped, and feet flat. From now on, all new techniques will include all previously learned techniques.

▶ **(2) Originate Body Turning from the Hip Fold: The Kwa**

The body has many natural hinges. The joints in your fingers allow the fingers to bend. The wrist joint allows the hand to bend; the elbow allows the arm to bend. In the hip, this hinge is located in the region around the inguinal groove which the Chinese call the kwa.

Most people turn to the side by using the muscles between the ribs and hip bone or, even more commonly, by turning their shoulders. From Chi Gung's point of view of body and spinal integrity, this type of turning is incorrect. The body should actually turn from the inguinal groove. Later, when that stabilizes, you can add the muscles of the waist, or *yao* in Chinese. Under no circumstances should you turn the waist using the shoulders, since this breaks the energetic connection between the arms and the spine, and twists the spine.

▶ **(3) The Hip Fold Leads the Spine, Waist, and Chest**

In the same way that you do not want to energetically dissociate the arms from the spine, you do not want to dissociate the spine from the hips, waist, and chest. To keep these connected, the movement must originate from the kwa, with the waist joining with the hip, and the chest then joining to the waist. Practice keeping this connection with the arms held forward as described in Exercise 1. There must be a straight line from the shoulder nest to the kwa on both sides. These four points must always remain in alignment to prevent the spine from twisting and to cause equal pressure on all the internal organs.

When turning, there is a tendency for the body to disintegrate. The legs will need to have their alignment checked, and the arms will again tend to deviate from parallel.

Even if these procedures seem simple, a good teacher is invaluable. You will find there is a great difference between what people think they are doing and what they are actually doing. A teacher can be a great help in pointing out discrepancies between the two.

▶ **(4) The Body Twist Massages the Organs**

The primary function of this turning from side to side (other than from learning to mesh the trunk, arms, and legs into one unit), is to pressurize the internal organs. Such twisting and wringing of the internal organs will bring them up to optimum condition in the same way that the twisting of a massage practitioner tones your muscles. The procedure described here causes chi to accumulate in the internal organs and will connect the spinal energy with the internal organs. This turning also automatically activates the chi flow in the "belt" meridians that wrap around the body.

▶ **(5) Shift Weight from One Leg to the Other**

In this exercise, the weight shifts from leg to leg as the waist pivots from side to side. In the middle position, the weight is evenly distributed on both feet and the waist is facing forward. Move the weight 100% to the left leg and turn the waist to the left. Move back through the middle position, and then move the weight 100% to the right leg as the waist is turning to the right. Repeat. (Many people will unconsciously tend to do the opposite: when turning to the right, they will keep their weight on the left leg.)*

Fourth Exercise: Sink One Side to Raise the Other

The next technique establishes a simple pumping action in the body, so that energy rises up one side of the body and drops down the other.

▶ **(1) Sink One Hand, Feel the Other Hand Rise**

Begin with one arm raised to shoulder level and the other at the side. Palms face toward the ground. As you lower one hand, the other simultaneously rises. The arm sinking downwards should create a feeling of energy or blood descending down the corresponding leg and into the floor. The sinking of energy down one side of the body should be felt to cause energy to rise up the other side, and lift the other hand up. As you practice this pulley action, it is imperative that the sinking hand cause the other

*Beginners will initially find it easier to first shift 100% onto one leg before turning.

hand to rise, and not the other way around. Energy sinking down the body will always cause energy to rise, while raising energy up the body may or may not cause energy to sink.

▶ **(2) Coordinate Sinking the Arm and Leg on the Same Side**

Next, shift the weight from side to side so that the leg receiving the weight is on the same side as the sinking hand—when the left hand is sinking the left leg is gaining weight, and vice versa. This will cause energy to rise up the opposite extending arm and leg.

Fifth Exercise: "Spinning Silk" with the Arms and Legs

▶ **(1) Chan Sz Jin: Spiral Energy that Gives Natural Power**

Now we're ready to discuss the spiraling of the arms. Natural joint movement and energy flow in human beings moves in spirals, similar to the structure of the DNA helix. Most people only use this spiraling action minimally, athletes use it more, and people with exceptional physical and movement abilities, who are able to keep these abilities into old age, use this spiraling action almost exclusively.

In Tai Chi Chuan, this action is called *chan sz jin*, or twisting silk, which is a metaphor for the way silk is spiraled out of the silk cocoon so that the threads don't break. In Hsing I and Ba Gua, this same idea is called *luo shuen jin*, or drilling or twisting strength, which is taken from the action of drilling a screw into a wall. The names are different but the function is the same. The twisting of the muscles, which follows the natural spiraling energy in the body, can be first observed in babies. The first attempt of babies at moving their arms and legs, at turning over and crawling, is done with spiraling movements, not straight line muscular movement.

▶ **(2) Practice Spiraling with the Entire Arm**

To learn to be aware of this spiral energy, we will first concentrate on the arms, and later add the waist and legs. Place the hands to the side, by your hips, with your fingers pointing straight ahead. The wrists are bent so that the palms and tips of the elbows face the floor and press slightly downwards. Beginning with the least coordinated arm, slowly and smoothly raise

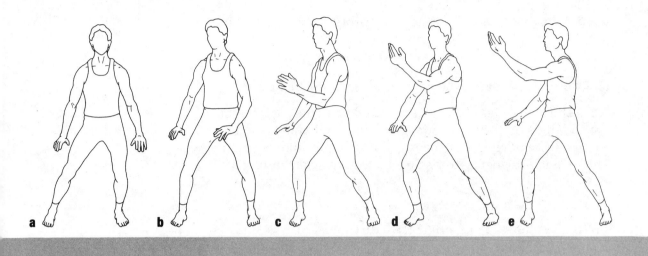

Figure 6-5 Cloud hands. This movement is a continuous flow. The positions shown are transitional guides, not static end points. (a) Starting posture: weight 100% on left leg, arms at sides (b), (c), (d), and (e) Shift weight to 100% on right leg, as the body turns to the right. Simultaneously, spiral and raise the left arm. (f) Begin to shift and turn to the left. Simultaneously, the upper arm begins to

and turn the hand, until it is at a height somewhere between the chest and nose. The higher your hand goes, the greater the stretch of your back and shoulder blades. Remember the 70% rule, and only increase the height of your hands as your back opens up. The hand ends on the centerline, with the palm facing upward at a 45° rounded angle, and toward the face. The arm then returns along the same circular path, ending in its original position.

As in all Taoist body practices, the spiraling of the arm begins at the space between the spine and shoulder blade, continues through the shoulder, upper arm, elbow, and forearm, and completes in the fingers.

The trick is to turn the hand exactly in proportion to the rate that the hand is rising or sinking, so that when the hand has risen 10% of the distance from hip to nose it has rotated 10%. At the midpoint from hip to nose, the hand would be vertical, or 50% rotated, and so on.

During this procedure, it is extremely important that the armpits are open and the arms and ribs do not touch. For women, it is very important to maintain, *at all times*, at least a distance the size of a fist between the breasts and the arms, especially the sides of the arms. Also, the elbow is always bent and

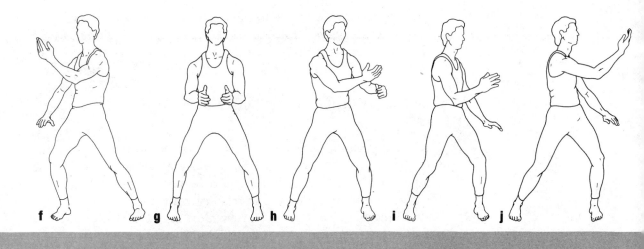

spiral and sink, the lower arm begins to spiral and rise. (g) Mid-point: weight
equally distributed on both legs, body faces straight ahead, palms face each
other on opposite sides of the centerline. (h), (i), and (j) Continue to shift and turn
until weight is 100% on left leg, body turned to left. Simultaneously, spiral the arms
until the left hand is palm down at side of hip and right hand is opposite the nose.

sinking downwards, so that at all times there would be room
for an egg or small orange to fit in the crook of the elbow. The
shoulders stay down while the arms rise.

▶ **(3) Coordinate the Arm Spiral with the Pivot in the Kwa**

The rising, falling, and spiraling of the arm is then joined with
turning from the hip and shifting the weight. As the waist turns,
the arm rounds and makes an arc to accommodate the turning of
the waist. The thumb finishes by the hip bone on the center line
of the side of the body, and the fingers point in the exact same direction as the groin. In fact, the groin, solar plexus, nose (head),
and fingers, as well as the four points of the kwa and shoulder's
nests, *point in the same direction at all times*. The side with the palm
pointing down is the side with the weight. Repeat the same procedure with the opposite hand and arm.

▶ **(4) Twist the Leg Muscles**

The thigh and calf muscles should twist in the same direction as
the waist, and at a speed proportional to that of the arm twist.
The twisting, or wrapping, of the leg muscles has two functions.

First, it prevents damage to the knee joint. Second, it spirals the tissue of the leg, so that the spiraling energy developed in the Spiraling Energy Body (another volume of this series—Advanced Chi Gung) can be more readily absorbed by the body.

▶ (5) Practice the Complete Cloud Hands Movement

The next step requires both hands to work simultaneously, which coordinates the left and right sides of the brain. With your weight completely on the left leg and your body turned to the left, your left hand will be palm down by the left hip and the right hand will be palm up in front of your nose.

Slowly begin to shift your weight to the right. When you reach the midpoint (i.e., weight 50/50, facing straight ahead), both of your hands will be at the same height, palms facing each other, near the centerline of the body. When you finish turning to the right, the left hand will be palm up at the nose and your right hand will be palm down at the side of the hip, below the armpit. Both hands will be rotating at a speed exactly proportional to the speed that they are rising and falling. With practice, Cloud Hands should become one smooth movement, rather than two separate movements on each side.

Though this exercise can be fairly difficult, it can also give the body a greater sense of freedom and energy than it has ever known before. This one simple Cloud Hands* movement is the foundation for almost every movement done in Tai Chi Chuan. The additional movements in Tai Chi forms just serve to increase the lengthening of tissue begun here. This lengthening or stretching opens up all the congestion in the body, increasing chi and loosening the body.

---

*The name "Cloud Hands" is not exclusive to Tai Chi. The author has seen over 400 exercises in China that use the name Cloud Hands, which is essentially a poetic term open to numerous interpretations.

CHAPTER 7

The First Swing

The Swings Energize Vital Organs and Joints

The next three exercises, called *swai shou* in Chinese (and generally referred to as "the swings" in English) have the basic function of energizing the upper, lower, and middle internal organs, as well as fully opening up the joints of the hips, shoulders, elbows, and hands.

The Three Tantiens *and Three* Jiaos *of Chinese Medicine*

From the point of view of practicing chi development, there are three main tantiens, each of which has a different function. The lower *tantien*, near the belly, is the source of life in the physical body. (This was discussed in Chapter 4.)

The middle tantien, located around the center of the sternum (i.e., the heart) is the energy center through which a person connects and forms relationships with other living things and their emotions, as well as being the source of thoughts and intentions. This is the source of compassion and benevolence, as well as the place where negative emotions are transformed.

The upper *tantien,* located at the third eye, is responsible for connections with discorporeal beings, subtle forms of thought, and other dimensions and places.

In terms of beginning Chi Gung, we are primarily concerned with the lower *tantien;* the upper *tantiens* are focused on in more advanced Chi Gung and Taoist meditation.

We are concerned with the three burners, or jiao, of the body. The lower jiao, which begins below the lower *tantien* and extends down to the floor, is primarily concerned with the functioning

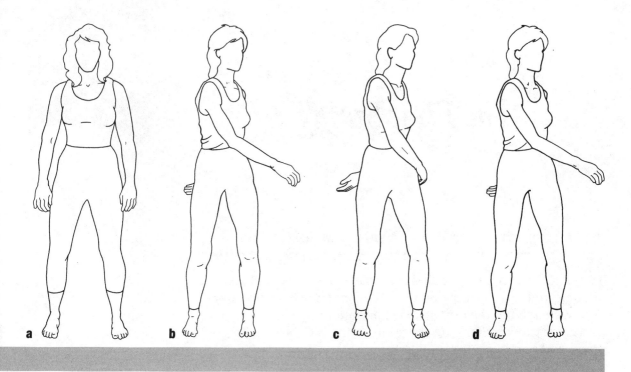

Figure 7-1 The First Swing. This movement is a continuous flow. The positions shown are transitional guides, not static end points. (a) Starting posture: weight equally distributed on both legs, body facing straight ahead, arms at sides. (b) and (c) Shift weight 100% to left leg and simultaneously turn to left; hands

of leg movement, urinary genital health, the large intestine, and the kidneys (which are also influenced by the middle burner).

The middle jiao extends from the *tantien* to the solar plexus and is responsible for the health of most of the organs—the small intestine, spleen, pancreas, liver, stomach, and gallbladder. The upper jiao extends from the chest to the top of the head, including the arms. It is responsible for the health of the heart, lungs, brain, and arms.

Each of the three swings energizes one particular burner. The First Swing has the primary function of opening the chi of the lower internal organs, the genital urinary area, the stomach, and the intestines. This swing will be of particular interest to people with constipation, sexual weakness, and kidney difficulties, both in terms of Western and Chinese medicine, and is particularly helpful for those who have cold and clammy hands and feet.

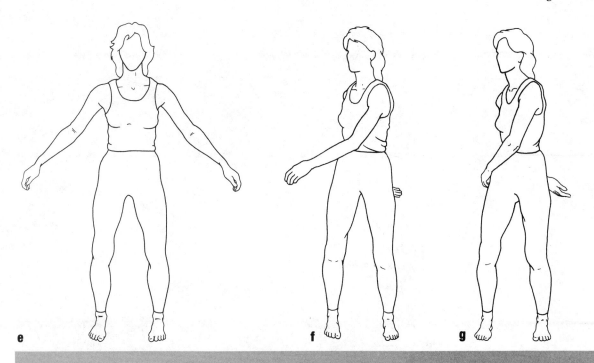

will swing in to touch body. (d) and (e) Begin to shift weight to the right and simultaneously turn back to mid-point; hands will swing out. (f) and (g) Shift weight 100% to the right and simultaneously turn to right; hands will swing in to touch body.

Instructions for the First Swing

Leg and Hip Movement Is the Same as Cloud Hands

The shifting of the weight, the opening and closing of the joints of the legs, the turning of the waist and the bending at the inguinal cut (kwa) are essentially the same as you learned before in Cloud Hands.

▶ **(1) Increase Speed of Twisting**

Now, however, the weight is shifted from leg to leg fairly quickly. Begin practicing the movement faster than slow motion and yet not as quickly as possible. It is extremely important that the head remain on the centerline of your body, along with the nose, the

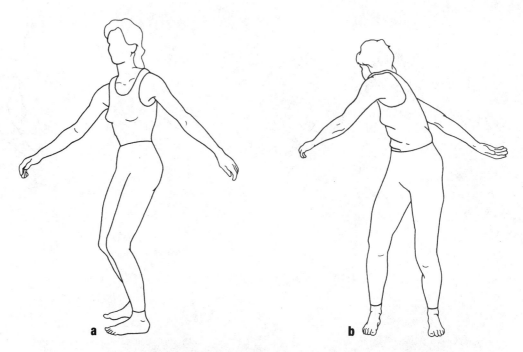

a   b

Figure 7-2 Maintaining integrity of centerline. (a) Correct: nose, solar plexus, and groin in a line. (b) Incorrect: Shoulders and head turned more than hips.

breastbone, the navel, and the groin, and that the four points of the shoulder's nest and kwa stay aligned (Fig. 7-2a).

▶ (2) Avoid Strain with the Proper Hip-Knee-Ankle Alignment

Though the legs are essentially the same as in Cloud Hands, it is worth re-emphasizing that the perineum must stay open, the body must turn by folding at the inguinal groove, the knees must be slightly bent (especially easy to forget with the weightless leg), the ankles and knees must be properly aligned, and the thigh muscles must twist in the same direction as the waist so that no strain is created in the lower back or the knees.

▶ (3) The Swinging Arms Must Be Totally Limp

The arms dangle from the shoulders, without using muscular control to move them in any direction. In other words, they should hang as though they were dead. Then use your awareness to make the shoulders, elbows, wrists, palms, and fingers as soft and relaxed as possible. With each swing, as the internal organs get warmed up, try to make the arms softer and softer until the joints of the arm feel as though they are filled with water or a soft warm liquid.

Practice "Arm Drops" to Release Shoulder and Elbow Tension

Particular attention must be paid to relaxing the elbow joints and removing any strength from them. To learn what it is like to have no strength in the arms, have someone hold your upper arm parallel to the floor, with elbow bent so that the forearm points to the sky. Relax the arm completely. The holder then lets go of the forearm, which should, if the elbow is relaxed, drop with the force of gravity. The habitual tension that most people carry in their arms usually does not let the arm drop. Practice this a few times until the arm falls down easily and comfortably, as a result of the release of all control and strength in the arm.

Next, raise the whole arm straight up and then let go. Repeat this until the whole arm can fall toward the floor in a relaxed manner, without any muscular contractions causing it to get stuck on the way down. Relaxation, increased circulation, smooth nerve flow down the arm, and an increase in chi will gradually allow the movements of this exercise to become smoother and smoother.

Power the Swing with Centrifugal Force

During the course of these swings, the arms will never act independently. They will simply be moved by the centrifugal force of the body as it swings to the left and right. Turning from the hips generates the force that moves the arms. A turn to the right side will bend the left arm toward the front of the body and the right arm toward the back of the body (Fig. 7-3). A turn to the left will do just the opposite.

As the centrifugal force swings the arms away from the body, the joints of the arms and shoulder open. As the centrifugal force swings the arms toward the body, the joints of the arms and shoulders close.

All of these actions must be accomplished by internal feeling, not looking. There is a great difference between intellectually knowing what your left and right sides are doing and

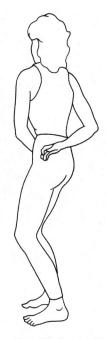

Figure 7-3 Turning to right propels right arm to back of body, left arm to front.

kinesthetically sensing what your left and right sides are doing. As mentioned before in the Cloud Hands section, it is preferable to work with a partner rather than rely on a mirror, as a mirror will provide only a visual/intellectual understanding.

It is of the utmost importance to begin to use awareness to relax and allow the elbow joint to let go. Under no circumstances should you move your arm muscles or bend the hands and arms. The shoulders should stay totally sunken and relaxed.

Hands Lightly Tap Kidneys and Abdomen

In the beginning, your arms will probably not bend higher than the top of your thighs at the end of your turn to the side. As relaxation of the arms and elbow joints increases, the arms will offer less and less resistance to the centrifugal force being generated by the turning of the waist. As this occurs, and as the turning of the waist becomes more and more fluid, the bend in the arms at the elbows will increase, until the forearms are eventually parallel to the floor. At this point, the hands will be *lightly* tapping the abdomen from the front and the kidneys from the back. Hitting the kidneys with excessive force is a sure way to hurt yourself, possibly even fatally. Kidney blows have been outlawed from boxing due to their danger, and though there are Chi Gung techniques for learning to absorb kidney punches, to learn such techniques requires the continued guidance of a master.

During the swings, it is extremely important that the space underneath the armpits stays open and the arms do not touch the ribs.

In time, with proficiency, as the arms come inwards they will bring healthy chi into the body, and as they swing away they will release stale or useless chi—in much the same way that oxygen is inhaled and carbon dioxide exhaled.

Do Not Drop Your Head

One of the most common mistakes made, which usually proves to be transitional, is that, as the practitioner relaxes the arms and waist more and more, the head drops down. For most people, the more they relax, the more the head tends to fall forward. This is a basic neurological reflex; as people go into a kinesthetic mode (i.e., feeling the body) the underlying tendency is for the eyes and head to drop and the spine to sag. During these exercises, it is very important to be aware of this tendency and correct it (keep your head straight up, your eyebrows and jaw parallel to the ground), so that the body is relaxed internally but does not collapse.

Keep Hands Soft

In this exercise, the arms and only the arms should collapse like a wet noodle, which brings us to the last detail: The hands must become totally soft, like a baby's. Avoid locking the fingers in any position, and keep the palms of the hands very soft and pliable. The amount of tension held in the hands indicates and affects the tension that is held in the rest of the body. Relaxing the hands will gradually spread relaxation throughout the whole nervous system.

The Core Energy

At this point, let's discuss an important aspect of the body's energy. There is a line of energy that runs vertically directly through the center of the body. A cut directly down the central axis of the body would bisect this energy core, which goes from the center of the head right down through the perineum, and continues through the center of the bone marrow of the arms and legs. This central vertical core of energy is the original energetic source of the formation of the human body from conception onward, manifesting in the development of the spine, the arms, and the legs, according to Taoist Chi Gung tradition. As you turn your body, you should keep your attention on your core channel and use it as the axis of your turn. However, you should also focus part of your attention on your lower *tantien* so that it is also the center of your turn. It is important that you move and turn equally from both places as this results in the largest output of energy to all the systems of the body. (This point also applies to Cloud Hands, but it is easier to learn to move from both places evenly here, in the swings, and then go back and include it in Cloud Hands.)

The Second Swing

The Second Swing Strengthens the Liver and Spleen, Dissolves Stress

The purpose of the Second Swing is to energize and strengthen the middle internal organs, including the spleen, liver, stomach, and pancreas, and the glands such as the adrenals. The footwork is essentially the same for the Second and Third Swings, though different from the footwork of the First Swing. The arm movements of swing one and two are essentially the same.

The Challenge: Shift Weight and Turn at the Kwa

The basis of all correct movement in Tai Chi Chuan, as well as in Hsing I and Ba Gua, involves physically and energetically joining the leg and waist together as the body shifts weight. This applies to any turning movement, any stepping movement, and any turns and dodges from side to side. The difficulty lies in getting the legs and waist to turn through sinking into, and expanding from, the inguinal cut (kwa), and not by twisting from the knee, which can slowly damage the lower back and leg joints.

Instructions for the Second Swing

▶ **(1) Feet Parallel, Shift Weight 100%**

Begin this exercise with your weight equally distributed on both legs, then shift your weight 100% to your right leg. With the hips

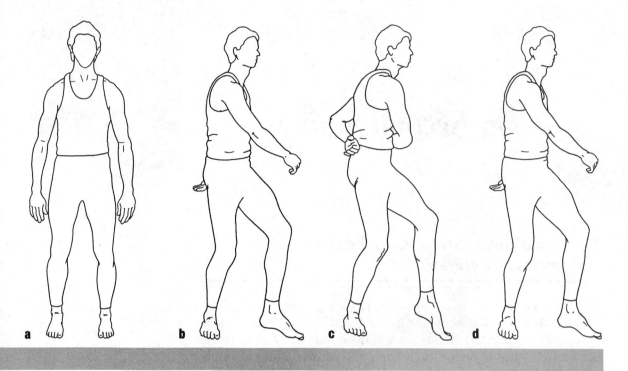

Figure 8-1 The Second Swing. This movement is a continuous flow. The postures shown are transitional guides, not static end points. (a) Starting posture: weight equally distributed on both legs, body faces straight ahead, arms at sides. (b) Shift weight 100% to right leg, begin to turn to left (allow left leg to pivot with the hip); arms will swing out. (c) Continue to turn to left (set down ball of left foot); arms will swing in to touch the body. (d) Begin to turn to right; arms

facing straight ahead, and feet in position for standing Chi Gung, lift up the left heel so that only the left toe is touching the ground. The foot, the knee joint, the crest of the pubic bone, the four points of the shoulder's nest and kwa, and the groin should all point in the same direction, that is, straight ahead. The feet should be exactly parallel.

▶ (2) As the Body Turns, Hip and Foot Pivot as One Unit

With the weight still on the right leg, begin to turn to the left, and let the left leg and foot pivot back to the degree that the hip turns. The more you turn a drafting compass, the larger the arc produced. Here, imagine the weighted foot to be the metal compass point placed on the paper. The spine and waist are the shaft of the compass. The bent left knee (not straightened at any point

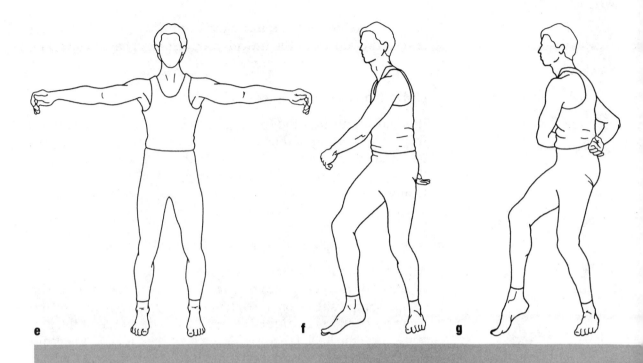

will swing out. (e) Mid-point: weight equally distributed on two legs, body faces straight ahead; arms are apex of extension. (f) Shift weight 100% to left leg, begin to turn to right (allow right leg to pivot with hip); arms will swing in. (g) Continue to turn to right (set down ball of right foot); arms will swing in to touch body.

during this exercise) is the connection between the shaft of the compass and the pencil, and the stable left ankle and foot are the pencil.

Suppose, for example, that the width of your hips is 18 inches. If your hips then turn 45 degrees, the toes of your left foot would move back in an arc of about 9 inches. Your left heel would also move back about 9 inches. This is only possible if the toes, ball of your left foot, the heel, the knee, the crest of the hip bone, the four points of the shoulder's nest and kwa, and the groin constantly remain aligned (pointing in exactly the same direction during the whole of the exercise), and if the bend of the left leg remains absolutely stable. The right leg neither straightens nor bends further.

The unweighted foot physically lifts an inch or two off the ground when you begin your turn, and the ball of your foot sets down on the ground at the end of your turning arc. This lifting and setting down of the unweighted leg is repeated as you go from side to center and center to side.

▶ (3) Do Not Turn Your Knees as You Pivot

It is important that the turning comes from the hips, and not from any twisting of the knee. As you rotate, turn the muscles of the calves in the same direction as the hips. This will prevent the torque created by the hips from pulling and twisting the knee in any direction. For people who enjoy skiing, this exercise will add to their skiing abilities considerably.

▶ (4) Pivot the Hip and Foot Back to Original Position

After turning completely to the left, turn back to the center, where your feet will again be parallel, heel off the ground. The weight should still be on the right foot. This is simply turning the compass back to its original point. Again, the angle of the ball of the foot, the heel, the knee, the crest of the hip, and the groin must remain perfectly aligned throughout the turn from the center to the side and from the side back to the center.

▶ (5) Shift Weight 100% and Pivot in the Other Direction

Put the heel down and simply shift the weight from the right to the left leg and do the same procedure to the left side. The entire sequence for the legs and weight shifting is as follows: from zero position, with weight at the center, shift the weight 100% to right leg; turn to the left as far as the hips will turn easily; return to zero position with the feet parallel, weight still 100% on the right leg. Shift all the weight to the left leg; turn hips to the right, turn back to center with the weight still on left leg. Then again shift to the right, and repeat continuously. Caution: If the weight is only shifted 50% when going to the side this can easily lead to knee strain. All weight shifts must be 100%.

The Arm Movements for the Second Swing

▶ (1) Concerning the Arms, the Second Swing Is the Same as the First Swing, with Higher Hand Level

The mechanics of the arm movements for the Second Swing are the same as those for the First Swing: The palm touches the front of the body and the back of the hand touches the back of the body. As your hips loosen and the arc of the hips increases, your hands will swing higher, eventually hitting between the navel and the solar plexus, where the middle internal organs are located.

▶ (2) Let Chi from Palms Penetrate to the Vital Organs

Touch the body very lightly in the beginning and, over time, slowly begin to tap the body harder, allowing the energy to penetrate deeper and deeper. At the beginning, the sensation from the hands will only be superficial, but eventually it will penetrate deep inside the body. Under no circumstances hit the body with any force or penetration in a spot where there is pain due to a malfunctioning internal organ or injury, and always tap the kidney area gently. If there is pain, touch the area as lightly as possible or even stop the hands just short of touching.

▶ (3) Spiraling Arms Circulate Chi

As the arms swing away from the body let them naturally twist so that the energy goes from the tantien up the spine, to the finger tips, and out into space away from the body. As the arms come in, energy from the air enters the body through the hands. This is another form of energy circulation, from center to periphery and from periphery to center. Now add this spiraling arm movement to the way you do the First Swing.

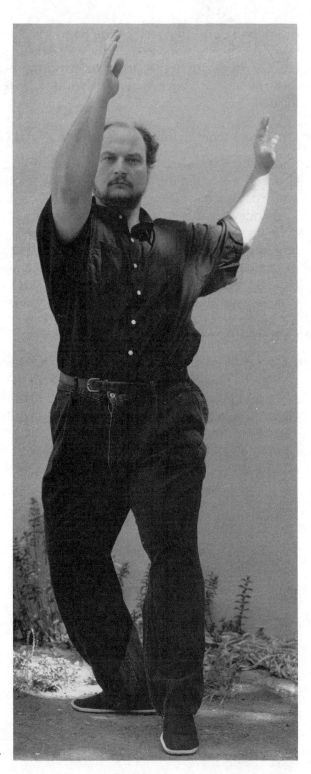

The author demonstrates the Third Swing.

CHAPTER 9

The Third Swing

The Third Swing Invigorates Chi in the Upper Body

The Third Swing has a number of functions. Most importantly, it works the upper internal organs (the heart and lungs) and it energizes the brain. Secondly, it adds spring to the vertebrae, so that they open and close with greater facility. Thirdly, it begins to open up the rotation of the shoulder joint, as well as the vertebrae of the neck, which are directly associated with the movement of the shoulders. Fourthly, it completely opens the hips and the kwa. Finally, the Third Swing teaches the body to instantaneously relax and let go on command. (Once an understanding of the body's energy has been gained through these Chi Gung exercises, it is possible to use the mind to direct the body so that movement is natural and effortless, not forced.)

Use More Pumping Motion in the Hip Fold Joint (Kwa)

The footwork of the Third Swing is essentially the same as for the Second Swing. Unlike the Second Swing, though, both the legs and the kwa open and close (bend and straighten). This pumps the synovial fluid in the hip joint, and releases a very powerful current of chi from the earth, feet, and legs that is pumped into the upper body organs, joints, spine, and brain.

Instructions for the Third Swing

▶ Shift Your Weight to Left, Center, and Right

Begin with your weight equally distributed on both legs. Bend and shift the weight to the right leg, and close the right knee and kwa while you pivot to the left, as in the Second Swing. When you've reached the end of your pivot, open the kwa but do not straighten the leg. Then close the kwa and bend both legs as you turn back to the center and a 50/50 weight distribution. At this point, open both the kwa and the knees, and straighten the legs. After this is completed, shift the weight 100% to the left leg and repeat to the right.

To close the kwa, squeeze down on the kwa muscles (this decreases the space between the vertebrae of the lower spine). To open the kwa, push or pump up the kwa muscles (this increases the space between the vertebrae). Alternating opening and closing the kwa activates the cerebro-spinal pump.

To open a joint, the space between the bones is enlarged. This usually, but not necessarily, results in the extension of the involved body part. To close a joint, the space between the bones is decreased.

The Third Swing Is, in Effect, a Four-Part Leg Exercise

(1) Weight 50/50 in center, both hips sinking

Begin with your legs evenly weighted, knees slightly bent, feet about shoulder width apart. Feel your body weight sinking easily through both legs from hip to ankle to earth.

(2) Weight 100% on right leg; right hip pivots open

Shift your weight 100% to your right leg, as the kwa and the legs bend (Fig. 9-1a). As you drop downwards, pivot to the left, as in the Second Swing, but also close your right knee and kwa. Both the left and right kwa open as you complete the pivot to the left, and the synovial fluid in each expands (Fig. 9-1b). It will take time for this movement to become fluid, as most people have let their pelvis "rust" and stiffen.

At the end of the pivot you open the kwa, but you do not straighten the leg—the right leg remains bent at the same angle.

(3) Weight 50/50 in center, both hips sink, legs bend slightly, then rise open

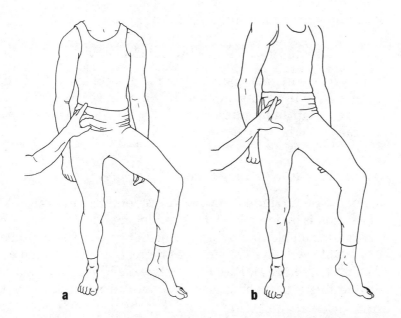

Figure 9-1 (a) Kwa closed (weight here is 100% on right leg). (b) Kwa open (weight here is 100% on right leg).

Closing the kwa and bending the legs again, pivot back to the center (Fig. 9-2a). When the weight is 50/50, open both the kwa and knees and straighten the legs (Fig. 9-2b). Feel the movement of energy moving from earth to feet to hips to upper body as you stand up. Most of the vertical movement upward should be caused by your kwa opening, not your knees.

(4) Weight 100% on left leg, left hip pivots open (step 2, opposite side). Repeat step 3. Repeat entire cycle.

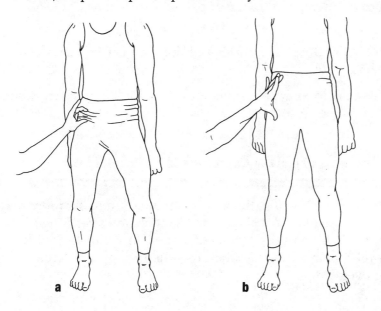

Figure 9-2 (a) Kwa closed (weight evenly distributed on two legs). (b) Kwa open (weight evenly distributed on two legs).

Guidelines for Practicing Leg Swings

▶ (1) Only Sink to 70% of Your Physical Capacity

By practicing in this fashion, your legs and knees will get stronger without risking damage. If you go lower than 70%, you may overstrain and injure yourself. Take it slow and easy, and gradually your body will soften up.

▶ (2) Knee Pain Is a Warning Signal

Any pain you might feel in your knees definitely indicates that a correction is in order. First, try standing higher, as you may be re-activating an old injury that you hadn't paid any attention to, or may not even have realized was there. Make sure when you sink that your knee and ankle are aligned and that you're turning your thighs in conjunction with your waist. Check that your lower back is straight. Make sure that the backs of both knees open on opening moves.

▶ (3) Feel the Chi Spiral Up Inside Your Body

Make sure that the turning in the third swing twists the lower internal organs and that this spiraling energy continues through the center of the body and up to the chest, lungs, neck, and directly into the brain. For purposes of this exercise, the brain will be considered part of the upper internal organs.

▶ (4) Make Sure the Pumping of the Kwa Is Clear and Deliberate

It's easy to forget about the kwa; we don't pay much attention to it in the West.

Preparatory Arm Exercises for Swing Three

In the Third Swing, the hands, shoulders, and shoulder blades are rotated to their maximum. As with any stretching exercise, it takes time to reach full extension, so we'll start with a few preliminary exercises before attempting the actual swing movement.

Exercise One: Rotate Arm and Shoulder

The footwork for this exercise is the same as for the Second Swing. With the weight on the left foot and waist facing to the right, place the left hand approximately shoulder height in front with the thumb facing the ceiling and the elbow bent. The tip of the elbow should point to the ground, and the arm should be extended and on the centerline of the body. The right arm and hand are held the same as the left—thumb up and shoulder height—and extended to the rear.

With the waist turned as far to the right as is comfortable, (remember to keep the head in alignment with the waist, with the nose, solar plexus, belly button and groin in a straight line, and to fold the kwa) slowly begin to rotate the hands. Maintaining the bend in the elbows, rotate the forearms so that the thumbs point to the floor, and then turn them back to their original position. Continue this until you have a clear sense of what it feels like for the forearms and upper arms to rotate, and especially what it feels like to have the thumb pointing straight up. Repeat this on the opposite side with the arms and legs reversed.

Exercise Two: Raise Arms and Let Them Fall Freely

Raise both arms over the head, palms facing out, and then let them fall. Do not throw the arms down, push them down, or force them down in any way. Just let them go completely, as if the strings of a puppet were cut. Release all control and let them drop naturally. An indication that this exercise is being done correctly is the sensation of the arms bouncing a little bit when they reach the bottom and naturally swinging back up. It's useful to practice this for ten minutes or more, unless you are very relaxed. If you are very tense, you may need to practice this particular exercise for several hours before progressing to the next section.

Exercise Three: Partner Tests if Your Arms Flop Freely

With your arms extended to the front, have a partner hold your arms at the wrist and forearm. Now release any tension in your

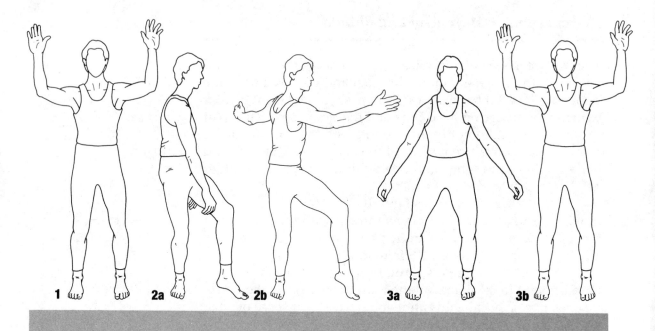

Figure 9-3 The Third Swing. This movement is a continuous flow. The positions shown are transitional guides, not static end points. Step 1: weight equally distributed on both legs; body faces front; arms up as shown. Step 2: (a) Shift weight 100% to right leg as you turn to left; simultaneously, sink in your kwa and drop your arms. (When you turn to the left, allow left leg to pivot with hip.) (b) Open kwa to propel arms up as shown. Step 3: (a) Simultaneously, shift weight so that it is evenly distributed on both legs, turn body to face front, sink in kwa and drop arms. (b) Open kwa to propel arms up as shown. Step 4:

arms, and have your partner bring your arms down to your side. Most people find it very difficult to release control of their arms, so have your partner move your arms an inch or two at a time at first and then gradually increase the distance, until he or she can freely and randomly move your arm anywhere from your head to your knees without any help or resistance on your part. Your entire arm should become a floppy dead weight.

After mastering this exercise, you should be able to raise your hands over your head and drop them below your knees in a totally relaxed fashion. For some people, it may take an hour or two to put this idea into practice. Tension is an easy habit to acquire. Once tension is accumulated and stored in the body it is difficult to release, but if you are gentle and patient with yourself, it can be done.

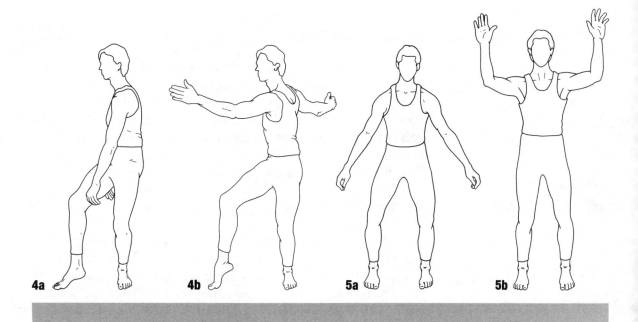

4a   **4b**   **5a**   **5b**

(a) Shift weight 100% to left leg as you turn to right; simultaneously, sink in kwa and drop your arms. (When you turn to the right, allow right leg to pivot with the hip.) (b) Open kwa to propel arms up as shown. Step 5: (a) Simultaneously, shift weight so that it is evenly distributed on both legs, turn your body to face front, sink in kwa and drop arms. (b) Open kwa to propel arms up as shown.

The Third Swing Is a Five-Part Movement

▶ Step 1: Facing Center, Raise Arms Above Head

Stand with the feet shoulder-width apart and parallel to each other, body facing forward. Raise both arms above your head, palms facing forward, fingertips towards the sky. The knees and kwa are open.

▶ Step 2: Drop Arms, Rotate Hips to Left, Swing Arms Up

Shift weight to the right leg and turn to the left, as you learned to do in the Second Swing. Simultaneously, let the hands drop, as though they had been held by puppet strings that were suddenly cut.

With all your weight on the right leg, arms facing downward, open your kwa and knee but do not straighten your leg. Allow the energy generated by the dropping of the arms and the opening of the kwa to lift the arms. Rotate the hands so that both are thumbs up, with the right hand on the center line in front and the left hand to the rear. Depending upon how much tension has been released from the arms, the degree of turn in the waist and hips, and especially on the opening of the kwa, the hands may finish anywhere from navel height to above the head. The height the arms raise is the height to which energy travels up the body. Do not force your arms upward—that will only stop the flow of chi. Just let them rise as far as they go without the use of muscular force.

Beginners will most likely be quite tense, and the arms will rise correspondingly little. With practice, and the gradual release of tension, the waist will turn more freely, the shoulders rotate more, the kwa open more, and the hands will go higher and higher, until they finally swing up in the air vertically. The legs go through a similar process, bending only slightly at first, but increasing until a deep squat is possible.

An important safety rule: When beginning this exercise, find out how far you can squat and turn, and then only squat and turn about half that amount. Slowly, over many weeks, increase to 70% of your capacity, but never exceed that amount. Westerners do not use squat toilets, so the ligaments of our knees are not very flexible. Therefore, it is prudent and vitally important that the strength of the knees be increased gradually. Under no circumstances, even if your body is very loose, exceed this 70% rule. This exercise includes a torquing action that has few western equivalents, so be slow, gradual, and gentle so that you do not hurt yourself by being overly zealous.

▶ Step 3: Drop Arms, Rotate Hips to Center, Swing Arms Up

Bring the legs back to parallel, weight 50/50, by closing the kwa and turning the waist back to the center. Drop the arms simultaneously.

Turning back to the center creates quite a bit of centrifugal force, and it is this force, in combination with the opening of the kwa and straightening of the legs, which raises the arms back to their original position. Once again, do not use any voluntary muscular lifting action. In the same way the arms are released to drop, they are released to swing back up.

As the body rises, the legs straighten, the kwa continues to lengthen, and the spine and neck raise. The arms rotate back to their original position, so that by the time the body finishes its motion the hands are shoulder-width apart with the palms facing forward and the fingertips lengthening out.

▶ Step 4: Drop Arms, Rotate Hips to Right, Swing Arms Up

Repeat—on the right side of the body, reversing the arm and leg positions—the same procedure described in step 2.

▶ Step 5: Repeat Step 3

Repeat the entire cycle.

Guidelines for the Third Swing

▶ (1) Rising and Sinking Opens the Macrocosmic Orbit

The lifting of the arms, the straightening of the spine, and the opening of the legs will cause energy and blood to rise up the body. The lowering and closing of the arms, legs, and waist will cause the energy and blood to move down. Together, these actions vigorously circulate the body's energy along what is called the large heavenly, or macrocosmic, orbit.

▶ (2) Hands Will Swing Higher with Practice

As practice increases the height the hands reach, different organs will benefit. When the hands reach the level of the heart and lungs it is these that will benefit, and as the hands ascend higher and higher, the energy will flow more and more into the brain.

▶ (3) Using Effort to Swing Arms Stifles Chi Flow

If, however, you use your volition to raise and lower the arms, the circulation of energy and blood to your spine, heart, lungs and brain will be only minimally increased. (You will only be doing a purely physical exercise, not one that will amplify your chi.)

▶ **(4) Lift Your Head Gently**

It is easy to let the head fall forward during this exercise. The head falling forward will tighten the neck and shoulders and impede the swinging of the arms. So remember to keep the head gently lifted off the spine.

CHAPTER 10

The Tai Chi Spinal Stretch

A Supple Spine Is the Backbone of Good Health

In many ways, the Tai Chi spinal stretch is probably the single most important technique in this book. In America, a medical problem that necessitates huge amounts of health care involves back and neck pain. Such pain may reflect prolonged deskwork time and/or enormous mental tension.

The spine stretch has as its goal the gaining of complete control over the movement of the spinal vertebrae. Practice of this exercise will ultimately result in the ability to move each and every vertebrae of the spine independently, and without relying on any external movement. This level of control is far beyond normal: Most people can barely feel their backs except when it aches. In fact, many people in America cannot even feel the muscles of their backs.

This technique has been used to help "incurably" bad backs, and can be done by anyone. People with severe back problems should use very small movements, and perhaps not even bend the spine at all at first.

The methodology of the spine stretch, which derives from classical Taoist body practices and which is integral to the performance of Tai Chi Chuan and the other internal martial arts, is quite different from the common back stretches found in any exercise or yoga class. Common back stretches essentially employ a rolling motion, where from a standing position the head and neck, then the chest, then the mid- and lower back, collapse as the upper body moves progressively closer and closer to the floor. This is the exact opposite of what you'll be doing in the Tai Chi Spinal Stretch.

The Spine Warmups

Spine Warmup 1: Lying on the Ground

Lie on the ground with your knees up in the air, so that the whole length of your back is more or less touching the ground. Begin to take very deep breaths, until it feels as if your breath is extending back to your kidneys. Take a few minutes, until you can use your breath to feel all the vertebrae along your spine. What we are attempting to do now is to get a sense of the difference between your back muscles and the vertebrae of your spine. By pressing up with your legs and lifting your bottom, or lifting up your head and neck and shoulders, you want to make each small section of your spine touch the floor in an isolated fashion, so that you can clearly differentiate the different sections of the spine. If you have a back problem do this on mats or thick carpet to protect your back.

Spine Warmup 2: Standing, Bend at the Kwa Only

Stand with the feet hip- or shoulder-width apart and keep your buttocks tucked under, so that your lower back is straight and your tailbone does not move backward.

From the kwa, and with the spine absolutely straight, bend over as far as possible. If you are very loose, bend until the spine is parallel with the floor; otherwise just go as far as is comfortable. It is important that the spine does not bend or twist in any way, so treat it as though it were a steel rod from the top of the neck to the tail bone, but *be sure not to tense the back muscles while doing this.* Raise up the same way, using the muscles of the kwa, again keeping the back straight with the tailbone unmoving the whole time. During this process, the feet do not move and the shins and thighs remain parallel to each other, with the perineum open. Keeping the feet still reduces the chance of the knees bowing out.

As you slowly go down from vertical, you want to make sure that the energy from your spine is going down your legs into the floor in an ever stronger fashion. Keeping your back absolutely straight, as you internally release each energetically bound vertebra, the energy released from each has to go down through your legs to the floor. (Use the dissolving technique you learned in Chapter 3 to accomplish bringing energy down to the ground.)

The purpose of this preliminary exercise is to make your legs and hips strong enough to support the weight of your back and neck, and to help your feet to gain the ability to root into the ground. In order to stabilize your balance, you will usually need to practice this warmup 10 or 20 times over a few days, or much time and energy will be wasted trying to maintain balance during the more complicated spine stretch itself. A half an hour to an hour of this preliminary warmup will save many hours of confusion, as well as prevent strain of the lower back.

Work with a partner, who will make sure that you are not arching or bending your back or neck in any way. Here again, it is very easy to feel as if you are not arching your back when in fact you are. Feedback from a partner can be very useful in this situation.

The Spine Stretch: First Half

Bending the Spine: Release Tension from Within

The critical component of the first half of the spinal stretch is the ability to put your mind inside your body and release any strength, tension, or chi blockage, as you let go of muscular volition and control of your back muscles. In other words, it is necessary to target your mind on a part of your body and then let go of all accumulated control or holding (i.e., dissolve the energy in each inter-vertebra space—"ice to water to gas").

A good way to get a feeling for what this is like is to hold your hand in a fist without squeezing or tightening it. Then mentally release everything that allows it to be in a fist until it opens, and then release all sense of physicality into the air away from your body. This can also be practiced by closing your eyes and relaxing them open, curling your toes and relaxing them open, etc. Become aware of the internal processes that allow this kind of relaxation to take place. At first, only use this technique on places that easily open and close and, at least initially, avoid places of chronic tension in your body, building successes in earlier places in your body before getting to the work you most need to do.

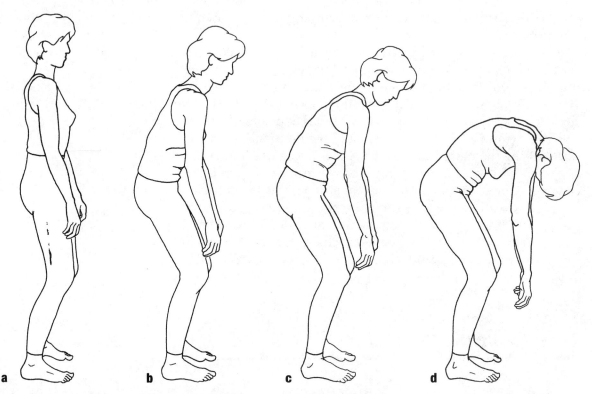

a   b   c   d

Figure 10-1 The Spine Stretch, first half. (a) Starting posture: feet parallel, back straight, head lifted, chest dropped, belly relaxed, shoulders rounded. (b), (c), and (d) Gradually release vertebrae from bottom to top, bending forward as each release is achieved. Release from the posterior (back) side of the vertebrae.

▶ **(1) Mentally Release Tension in the Vertebrae at the Base of the Spine, from the Posterior (Back) Side of the Vertebrae**

Stand with the feet between hip- and shoulder-width apart, whichever is the most comfortable. Begin by mentally releasing all the tension between your sacrum and your fifth lumbar vertebra. It is actually possible to slightly separate the theoretically immovable bones of the sacrum, but this is a more advanced practice. Keep the back straight above the next vertebra up. Do not release the tension found above the fifth vertebra—let it remain there for the moment. After releasing the tension between those vertebrae (that is, increasing the space between the vertebrae thereby taking the pressure off the disc) gently incline the hips slightly forward. When you incline your hips slightly forward, gravity pulls these first vertebrae slightly apart.

Now, your body may be so bound up that it takes a few weeks before you get an actual physical separation of the vertebrae, but you must continue to work on this area with your mind until some sort of release is felt in the nerves or chi. Over time, the release of the nerves will cause the muscles to let go and allow the vertebrae to separate slightly. In order for the body to bend at all, the vertebrae must release and separate on some level, although it can be so slight as to be unnoticeable—what we want to do here is increase this stretch.

▶ (2) Release and Stretch Each Vertebra, One at a Time

Next, move to the area between the next two higher vertebrae and release. Once the release is felt, bend forward ever so slightly, so that gravity will increase the distance between these two vertebrae: the degree of release will increase with time. Again, above these vertebrae, nothing moves, bends, or twists in any fashion.

It is very helpful to have a partner place their finger(s) on the vertebra you are trying to release. As most people have a poor sense of their backs, this helps you direct your attention to the appropriate vertebra. It is a good idea to begin by releasing a few vertebrae at a time, eventually fine tuning your sensitivity to the point where you can release one vertebra at a time.

Continue this process, releasing one vertebra (or group of vertebrae) at a time. Every time you release a vertebra you may further release any of the vertebra below it, but you must keep bound and unmoving the vertebrae above the one you are working on. As you approach the neck, it will be very difficult to keep the head from flopping. Be aware of this tendency, and have a partner help you correct this by holding his or her arm in front of your nose. Your partner will immediately let you know when you have bent your upper spine and neck prematurely.

▶ (3) Progressively Release the Shoulder/Arm Joints as You Release the Cervical Vertebrae

Releasing from the big vertebra at the bottom of the neck (the seventh cervical) through to the atlas (the first cervical) proves to be the most difficult for the majority of people. When releasing from the seventh to the first cervical vertebrae, also begin to progressively allow the joints of the shoulders, elbows, wrists, palms, and fingers to open up, and continue this opening as you progress through the neck. By the time the atlas has released, the arm joints (to the fingers) should also be completely released.

▶ (4) Release the Skull Plates

After releasing the atlas, to the best of your ability begin to release the skull plates. The human skull is not one bone, but rather a number of plates joined together by sutures. These plates are capable of being released through voluntary action. When the spine, neck, and skull plates release, the nerve and chi flow in the body, as well as the strength of the cerebro-spinal pump, will be greatly improved.

Remaining bent forward, you will usually want to release energetically from bottom to top again. This ultimately culminates in waves of chi going up your spine to the top of your head and through your arms to your finger tips.

Raising the Spine to Strengthen It

The spine has basically two functions in a human being. One is to bend and flex (which has been covered in the first part of this exercise). The second function of the spine is to lift, so that we may stand erect. It is this second function that is addressed in the second half of the spinal stretch.

The Spinal Stretch: Second Half

▶ (1) Open and Lengthen the Anterior (Front) Side of the Spine as You Unbend

At this point, your legs are still shoulder-width apart and your spine, head, and arms are totally released. Again, *work from the bottom toward the top*, leaving the vertebrae above the area of focus unchanged. However, rather than releasing the spine at the lowest two vertebrae, allow them to lengthen and move apart, so that the distance between the vertebrae increases even further. This additional separation of the vertebrae causes a local lifting, or opening, of the body. In the first half of the stretch, the back of the spine is especially lengthened. In the second half, as you are coming up, it is the inner or anterior side of the spine that is especially lengthened and focused upon.

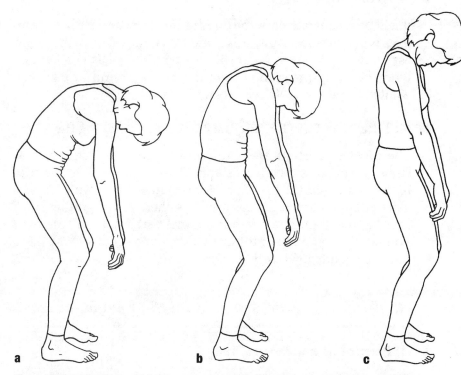

Figure 10-2 The Spine Stretch, second half. (a) Posture upon completion of first half (you are bent all the way forward). (b), (c), and (d) As you stand erect, open the anterior (front) side of the spine from bottom to top. Opening means lifting each vertebra in the front (vertebrae are already opened in back from the first part of the stretch).

▶ **(2) Unbend the Spine, One Vertebra at a Time**

Proceed to the next two higher vertebrae with your mind, and lengthen those straight up, leaving from the third vertebra to the top of your head still totally released and floppy. Again, it is very useful to have a partner put a finger between the two vertebrae you are working on, so that the area concerned can be felt more easily and more awareness can be brought to it. Your partner also will want to keep a hand on the back of your neck to stop your upper back and neck from straightening before their time. These must remain completely floppy and released, just as in the first half of the exercise your partner kept a hand in front of your nose to keep your neck and upper back from relaxing before their time.

▶ **(3) Avoid Stiffening the Neck**

It will be when you reach the middle of the upper back that problems will almost certainly arise, and the neck will have the greatest tendency to stiffen and raise or bend back. This is where, when bending the spine forward, your neck and upper back wanted to prematurely release downward.

▶ **(4) Take Extra Care Raising the Neck and Stretching the Skull**

The most important areas to consider are the opening and straightening of the vertebrae at the base of the neck to the base of the skull, and the opening of the plates of the skull. Paying extra attention to these areas prevents energy from getting stuck in the spine. From the seventh cervical vertebra to the plates of your skull, you will simultaneously want to gently push open your arm joints to your fingertips.

Guidelines for Practicing the Tai Chi Spinal Stretch

▶ **(1) Practice with a Partner First**

Your partner's hands on your back will help you begin to feel each vertebra of the spine as a separate entity.

▶ **(2) Learn to Separate Groups of Vertebrae, Then Individual Ones**

When you work by yourself in the beginning, it is quite natural to only be able to feel large parts of your back as a unit. For most people, the unit of sensation is anywhere from four to six vertebrae, though within a year most people are able to feel their vertebrae one by one. So at first, just release and open whatever your unit of sensation is; be it one, two, four, or even eight vertebrae.

▶ **(3) Maximum of Three Spinal Stretches per Practice Session**

Under no circumstance do more than three spine stretches in any one practice session. This is a safety precaution against overstraining. Also, after three spine stretches, the time/energy cost effectiveness of doing more spine stretches radically diminishes. If you feel as though your spine really wants a good workout, simply spend more time on each spine stretch rather than increasing the number of repetitions. You could also practice more than one session a day as long as there is a four-hour interval between sessions.

▶ (4) Avoid Sudden Increases in Practice Times

If you practice these exercises every day or every other day, which is the most beneficial way to do them, and for some reason your life situation prevents practice for a week or so, do not try to make up for lost time. Do a little bit less than you were practicing before your layoff. Increase incrementally with each practice session. In this way, you won't jar your nervous system or overstrain your muscles.

▶ (5) Focus on Releasing Chi, Not on Stretching

It is important to realize that it is not a requirement of the spine stretch to bend very low. What is important is the amount of nerve action through the vertebrae and how much chi is released in the spine. This is not a high school gym exercise. And again, make sure not to overstrain or fight through an injury—dissolve and melt the injury and tension away. You want your spine to regain the soft, natural flexibility of a child's spine, but this process takes time and can't be rushed.

Afterword

An Abundance of Chi Is Your Birthright

People in the Orient have developed methods that allow a human being to have tremendous vitality well past the point that the body is naturally overflowing with energy. Many of the practices developed in China have been kept secret for centuries, but I believe that now it is time for all human beings to have the chance to benefit from this profound life-serving knowledge.

From the ancient Taoist point of view, the vast majority of human beings are given plenty of energy at birth. At some point, though, if one has not lived a completely natural and healthy life (which is getting progressively more difficult all the time) this energetic abundance begins to fade, and more energy must be earned. A young blade of grass, a seedling tree, and babies are soft and flexible. With the coming of old age, the blade of grass hardens and can be easily snapped; the tree becomes brittle and dry; and elderly human beings stiffen until they can barely move.

You Must Practice to Reap the Benefits

Abundant life energy, the ancient Taoists observed, came with softness and pliability. The Tai Chi Core Exercises herein provide the foundation necessary to regain these qualities, but this path does require time and effort. It's your life and only you can determine your priorities. While the intellectual information in this book may be interesting in itself, the real value of this book can only come through the practice of these exercises. The proof is in eating the pudding, not in reading about what it tastes like.

Those who are thinking of learning Tai Chi Chuan or any internal martial art will find that learning and practicing these Core Exercises will increase their learning speed dramatically. I have personally seen, in the United States and Europe, many people who have practiced Tai Chi Chuan for ten or fifteen years and yet are not familiar with the basic principles involved with the Core Exercises—principles they should have learned from their teachers in the first year of practice. If anyone is thinking of learning Tai Chi or the internal martial arts, this is the best foundation possible.

For average people, who do not want to get into the complicated movements of Tai Chi but want to gain a significant number of the mental and physical benefits available from Tai Chi, these Core Exercises are perfect. Later, if they find these benefits really inspire them to learn Tai Chi, Hsing I, or Ba Gua, they will begin from the best possible starting point and will be far ahead of most beginners.

Appendix A
Guidelines for Practice

▶ **(1) Practice Until Your Joints Feel Well-Lubricated**

Often, individuals will reach a point in standing where they feel they have had enough—the body wants to move. At this point, begin Cloud Hands. Continue Cloud Hands until the contraction and stiffness of the body begins to go away and the major areas of immobility loosen up. (This activity can be thought of as the dry areas inside the body becoming wet and lubricated, especially your joints, hips, spine, and waist.) When the body begins to feel oiled, go on to swing one. Repeat this process through each of the swings—when "oiled" by one swing, proceed on to the next. After becoming proficient in these exercises, most people find that three to five minutes of Cloud Hands and one to two minutes of the swings is enough. The more time spent on each swing, the more lubricated the joints will become (up to a point, of course).

▶ **(2) If You Feel Pain, Use Slower and Smaller Movements**

If for some reason a pain comes up as a result of overstrain, simply go on to the next swing. The primary rule in these exercises is to do no harm to your body.

Now, a distinction must be made between the natural strain of exercise or stretching and the pain of damage. Pain in any of the joints means you should back off and review the instructions on how to do the exercise. If the instructions are being followed correctly and you get pain in a joint—whether elbow, knee, shoulder, or wrist—you could be overstraining yourself or opening up an old injury. In either case, moderate the range and pace of your movements, and if the pain continues beyond the mild stage, switch into the next swing. If it persists into the next swing, decrease your range of motion until the pain stops. Under no circumstances should you attempt to "work through" the pain of your joints. This same rule applies when you practice Tai Chi Chuan, Hsing I, or Ba Gua, or, for that matter, any internal exercise.

The soft tissue of the body is another matter. The small motions of Chi Gung may lead to burning or knifelike feelings in the soft tissue. The School of Hard Knocks invariably teaches most people what is meant by overdoing it in this regard. If the pain is severe, unless you are under the guidance of a master, back off. All athletes must learn to recognize their limits, and if you do not have much experience, it is best to err on the side of caution. Slight pain in the soft tissue is quite normal; a lot of pain is best avoided.

Most people do not know their limits, and consequently overdo it. This is particularly true of weekend athletes. While overdoing for a few seconds will not cause much damage, really pushing it for longer periods of time and over many days certainly will. Of course, the amount of strain a given individual can bear depends on many factors, such as age, weight, body type, and previous training.

▶ (3) Special Warning: Do Not Overstrain Knee Joints

Overstraining muscles will at worst result in a pull; the vast majority of people will stop well before that stage due to the pain involved. A pulled or overstrained muscle will heal within a few days, a few weeks, or, at worst, in a few months. On the other hand, tendon, ligament, or joint damage can last a lifetime and even require surgery. Be gentle with your joints—they are not replaceable. Muscles grow back, but joints do not.

For most people, pain in the knees or ankles means they need to stand a little higher. I really want to caution Westerners in general that they live in an upper-body culture, with concomitantly poor awareness of the joints in the lower body. In martial arts, this lack of awareness all too commonly leads to knee problems. The internal martial arts are known in China for their ability to heal back and joint problems. If you strain your joints, however, the twisting actions can easily weaken already weak structures and aggravate old injuries. These exercises can be of tremendous benefit if done correctly, but, like any type of exercise, they can also damage people who try to be heroes and go beyond their limits.

▶ (4) Movement Artists: If You Feel Fatigue, Change to the Next Swing

Obviously, people involved in movement arts will only be satisfied with the greatest possible range of movement. This desire will cause them to want to go beyond getting the joints lubricated to a sense of the joints dissolving and even a feeling of bonelessness. When this feeling is achieved, you are ready to switch to the next exercise. This is very difficult to put in terms of time, as it is possible to do Cloud Hands or each of the Swings as much as an hour (or two, or three) at a time. This is very individual, and only in a face-to-face encounter with a highly skilled instructor can exact parameters be stated. As a general rule, however, if fatigue begins to set in at one of the joints, it is time to move on to the next exercise. The trick is to optimize the amount of energy running through the system, without going over the line to exhaustion. This can only be done through self-observation, which leads to the direct understanding and experience of the limits as well as the strengths and possibilities of your body and mind.

▶ (5) Martial Artists: Don't Visualize Fighting Applications

For the martial artist, the previously discussed exhaustion and joint strain issues also apply. Additionally, martial artists tend to visualize all sorts of fighting applications, as these are inherent in the exercises. The tendency is to get so wrapped up in martial arts applications that the body's limits are forgotten, either intentionally or unintentionally. Try to avoid this mistake, for as well as damaging the joints it can create mental tension around the fighting techniques.

▶ (6) Best Time to Practice

As with most energy development exercises, the best time to practice begins about two hours before dawn, which is when the earth is most quiet and psychic disturbance is lowest. Another good time is early in the morning, around sunrise. Practice in the morning is best on an empty stomach, so that the energy of the body is not being dissipated by digesting breakfast. Have breakfast afterwards.

Early evening is also a good time, though one should avoid exercising too close to bedtime, as these practices generate energy.* If you do practice before going to bed, do swing one, then the spine stretch, then swing one again, this time doing it so that you actually feel as if you are falling asleep on your feet—let all your remaining tension fall into the ground. And for night owls, the period between 12 and 3 A.M. is actually quite favorable; here, too, the stresses and psychic disturbances generated by city life have begun to wind down. During these hours, the body is also naturally beginning to fill up with yang chi, and practicing Chi Gung will accelerate this process. Night owls normally lose yang chi by not sleeping during these hours; the practice of Chi Gung during these hours mitigates this problem. This is the perfect practice time for people who work the swing shift.

▶ **(7) "How Often Should I Practice?"**

(a) General public: a minimum of three to five times a week.

The first question on people's lips usually has to do with how much or how often to practice these exercises. For the first three years, it is strongly recommended to practice these exercises for a minimum of 10 to 20 minutes per session at least three or four times a week. Daily is best.

(b) Martial artists: daily

If you are practicing Tai Chi Chuan or other internal martial arts, after about three years you will have the sensitivity to work out your own practice session, but ideally these exercises should be done every day. Use all these exercises as a warm-up before your main workout, and use the swings and the spine stretch as an excellent wind down. Employed for these purposes, the swings only need to be done for two or three minutes.

(c) Runners and athletes: warm up and cool down

People involved in activities such as running or competitive sports will find that the swings and the spine stretch are excellent ways to release the stress and chi blockage that can occur after competition. These exercises will improve your recovery time dramatically. And they help loosen and lubricate the body prior to activity.

(d) Office workers: lunch and short breaks

It is exceedingly useful for people in high stress jobs to do the swings and spine stretch for a few minutes during coffee

---

*An excess of energy can keep you awake longer than desired much in the manner that strong coffee can.

breaks, when they are first feeling stressed, but before the stress has had a chance to settle in. A minute spent getting rid of stress at this stage can be incredibly valuable. The swings are recommended when there is only a minute or two to do something.

▶ (8) Use Chi Gung to Manage Stress

For people involved in high-stress jobs, it is important to understand how stress works. Stress begins with overexcitement of the nervous system and then slowly works its way deep into the body. It begins as wet cement, so to speak, and when the stress is prolonged this begins to harden (i.e., the contraction and constriction of the nerves and organs starts to become permanent). The stress of the morning begins to harden around lunch time. The stress accumulated after lunch will begin to set by evening or the end of the work day.

Five minutes spent doing the swings or Cloud Hands during a coffee break in the morning or the afternoon can prove to be of great value, in effect wiping away the day's stress and keeping the metaphorical cement wet. Ten or fifteen minutes at lunch can bring back the freshness of the morning. Practice after work can take away all the stress ("wet cement") accumulated during the day.

So far we have only discussed getting rid of the stress accumulated during the day. Any practice above and beyond this initial stress release will increase your core energy reserves, which your body/mind uses in times of crisis, emergency, or recovery from illness or accident. This core reserve of chi will also determine the quality of energy available later in your life.

▶ (9) Toxin Release Will Be Followed by Energy Flow

It needs to be kept in mind that in the early stages of practice (the first few months), these exercises cause the body to release a tremendous amount of stored toxins, which can result in feelings of fatigue, discomfort, and an unwillingness to practice. Toxins are released through the sweat, urine, and feces, and in the beginning you may notice that your sweat smells quite foul. This will pass, and soon your sweat will be relatively odorless.

While not a substitute for fasting and other cleansing methods, the Core Exercises, and the internal martial arts in general, are good adjunctive cleansing therapies. Once the initial layers of toxins and trapped energy are released, the energizing effects of these exercises will begin to be felt twenty-four hours a day.

Special Note for Women: Chi Gung causes increased blood circulation. Thus, during the menstrual cycle, Chi Gung practice may cause excessive menstrual bleeding. The Chinese medical view is that, if your menstrual bleeding is in fact increased during Chi Gung practice, you should reduce practice time or cease practicing altogether until your period is over.

Special Note for Men: Unless you have learned to regulate the internal flow of your Chi during sexual intercourse and control your ejaculations, it is best to avoid practicing Chi Gung two to three hours before and after intercourse. This avoids unbalancing the regulated flow of Chi gained through Chi Gung practice and prevents excessive energy loss.

Appendix B
Searching for
a Qualified Teacher

Instructions in Chi Gung must be followed accurately, and especially in the early stages of learning, it is important to have access to a competent teacher, so that in the small number of cases where problems arise, help is not far away. The instructions given in this book with regard to chi movement, rather than body mechanics, are not meant to be learned solely from this book. They are meant to enhance understanding while one is under the guidance of a qualified instructor.

The teacher needs to demonstrate to the student verbally, nonverbally, and by the quality of his life, what it is that the student is trying to do. If the teacher's chi is not full, if the teacher is not essentially relaxed, then it is highly unlikely that the student's chi will become full and relaxed. Chi Gung is not the acquisition of intellectual information, but is the process of becoming something. The person you model yourself after will also be imparting his or her energy to you. The quality of that person's energy will determine what you will get from the interaction.

In China they put it very simply: This kind of subject can only be learned from somebody who has got it. Many forms of athletic or intellectual skill can be learned from a good coach who is a poor practitioner. However, in chi development, the level of the teacher's accomplishment determines his capacity to transmit this development to the student. Ideal teachers are those whose personal chi is highly developed, as is their capacity to communicate to the student. As the old saying goes, "Some people can teach, some people can do, and those who can do both are very rare."

Do not be misled by a good pitch, for the words of chi development are very cheap, and anyone can say them. Also, be aware that an Oriental ethnic origin is no guarantee of expertise. Take your time, and check out all the teachers in your area (if there are any). Only learn Chi Gung from someone you sense is on the up and up. It might be better to wait than get involved in Chi Gung with somebody you are unsure of.

In the United States and Europe, at this moment, only a minority of the instructors would be considered competent by generally recognized traditional standards in China—standards which have been established over thousands of years of consistent experimentation and bitter experience. Though these traditional standards commonly do not guarantee fast and easy results, they generally allow students to reach their goals with sufficient effort and practice.

What to Look for in a Good Teacher

When considering Chi Gung teachers, the first questions to ask are: Have they been doing the type of chi work they are asking you to do for a minimum of ten years? Did they really understand their teacher's transmission, especially if their teacher did not speak the same language? Do they seem fairly well balanced psychologically? (If they are essentially open-minded, open-hearted, and generous of spirit, then you have a much better chance of getting the story straight. If they are not, and use information as a carrot to entice you, their neuroses may keep them from giving out the real stuff.) Look for mental and emotional clarity and physical well-being in a teacher.

Unfortunately, even if they do meet the above criteria, they may not know enough to debug their system if something goes wrong. Look for brutally honest and scrupulous teachers who have studied many systems completely and understand how they interface, or at the very least, know their own system down to the finest details. So that, if problems do occur, they are competent and willing to work with you to overcome your difficulties. Many Chinese learned as youngsters and teach adults, not realizing that the process of learning is different for children as opposed to adults.

Talk to ongoing students of a particular teacher to get a picture of what their practice is like; find out if they are getting something you would like to have. As the years pass, more and more Americans will be able to discriminate between good and bad Chi Gung, and you will be able to consult with them about what is going on.

Appendix C
The Importance of
Correct Chi Gung Practice

The vast majority of the thousands of Chi Gung techniques, including those found in this specific Chi Gung series, are health-supporting and safe. However, like any powerful tool, if used incorrectly, Chi Gung can cause damage as well as benefit. There are literally hundreds of Chi Gung practices that can cause significant problems, and it would be impossible to mention every one. Here I will endeavor to give the reader a healthy respect for the power of Chi Gung techniques and some means to discern which techniques are safe and effective.

Every Body Is Different

Humans have different levels of tolerance to stress and pressure. Some lead completely dissolute lifestyles and live long, healthy lives, while others live as purely as possible and live short, miserable lives. The difference lies mainly in the amount of energy they were born with and the strength of their nervous systems.

From the Chinese point of view, the capacity to bear stress is a function of the strength of the nerves. When the stress level surpasses the central nervous system's capacity to handle it, the nerves begin to break down, which results in all sorts of physical, emotional, and mental disturbances, and can eventually lead to organ malfunction and premature death.

Chi Travels through the Nerves

Since different people have nervous systems of different strengths, it is important that Chi Gung practices take this difference into account. Just as a lifestyle that some thrive on would send others to an early grave, so some Chi Gung systems that are fine for some are actually quite dangerous for others.

Chi travels through the nerves, and consequently it is the nerves that are potentially most at risk from incorrect Chi Gung practice. While proper Chi Gung practice strengthens the nerves, improper techniques can overload them, leading to the breakdown of all body systems.

Every message from the brain to the body, and vice versa, goes through the central nervous system. When practicing direct manipulation of the central nervous system, three precautions must be taken: (1) practice must be done within the proper limits, or the nerves will be damaged; (2) new pathways must lead to health and well being, not towards illness; and (3) the body must have enough time to balance out all these new inputs, so that the signal does not get scrambled—going too fast can cause serious problems for both the mind and body, as well as lead to hallucinations (imagining things are happening when they are not).

It has been proven consistently in China that Chi Gung, if practiced correctly, can bring about a reversal of internal organ malfunctions and can relieve all manner of stress by increasing the strength of the nerves. If done incorrectly, however, it can instead actually increase stress or damage organs. Just as a mechanic, using the same tools, can damage a car as easily as fix it.

Safety Comparison of Pranayama and Chi Gung

"Prana" in Sanskrit and "chi" in Chinese can both be translated as "the breath of life." The classical Yoga texts, when discussing Pranayama (energy development), always state that the most important requirement for learning is the guidance of a competent teacher on a frequent, preferably daily, basis. This requirement is based on the following presuppositions:

(a) Pranayama is inherently dangerous
(b) to avoid pitfalls, it must be practiced correctly

(c) if for some reason problems arise, the teacher must be on the spot to correct them before it is too late

(d) signs too subtle for a novice to notice will arise before problems develop. (Slight calibrations at this stage can mean the difference between learning correctly and self-injury.)

Pranayama Is Based on Breathing and Packing

Pranayama utilizes techniques that close down energy in one part of the body and build it up (pack it) in another. These techniques involve postures and the use of the breath.

As such, pranayama is an extremely precise science. Just as in a nuclear reactor it is crucial to develop exactly the correct amount of heat and pressure, so it is in Pranayama—and on an individual level the consequences of incorrect practices can be devastating.

In the West, as well as India, many people who practice pranayama techniques incorrectly suffer from physical and psychic problems as a result. Much of this is simply the result of a lack of competence on the part of the teacher, though it also can come from a frivolous disregard for what the teacher taught. And in America, especially, there are those who learn only from books. Such people do not have any way to be aware of potential problems, to know how much is enough, and to recognize what practices require the guidance of a teacher.

Pranayama Works Too Well

The difficulty with Pranayama practices lies not in the fact that they don't work, but rather that they work too well. If a technique has power, its power to benefit life is sometimes matched by its power to destroy it when practiced incorrectly or by a person of the wrong constitution.

Benefit-to-Risk Relationship in Chi Gung

In the Hatha Yoga Pranayama systems, which have the ability to initiate and carry through the genuine Kundalini process to self-realization, the potential benefits are roughly equivalent to the potential risks. In Chi Gung, however, the relationship between risk and benefit is more complex—some systems have low benefits and high risks, some average amounts of each, and some, like the techniques discussed in this series of volumes on energetics, have very low risks and high benefits.

Learning Chi Gung in China

Even in China it is very difficult to find a good Chi Gung teacher. Most teachers impart only one system, and teach that system as they learned it—by rote. They have no basic understanding of how it works and how it fits into the overall picture of Chi Gung.

The Chinese make a great distinction between people who know some Chi Gung techniques and people who are Chi Gung masters. This distinction is much like that between a computer operator and a computer programmer. The former knows how to push the buttons to make the system work, but doesn't know what to do if something goes wrong, or how to modify the system for specific needs. On the other hand, the programmer, or computer master, knows how to get the "bugs" out of the system should they appear, and how to adjust the program for a specific application or a particular user.

Students rarely investigate different Chi Gung systems before beginning to practice one, and once they have begun one with a given teacher, it is considered disloyal to even visit other teachers. Their teacher's word becomes gospel. This climate makes it hard for Chinese students to become expert in more than one branch of Chi Gung.

Taoists Stress the Spiritual Framework of Chi Gung

China is the oldest continuously civilized culture on Earth, and the Chinese are incredibly proud of that fact. Historically, they have considered themselves the only civilized nation on Earth. When this attitude is combined with the memory of how poorly Westerners have treated them in the past, it is understandable that many Chi Gung masters do not want to have anything to do with foreigners, and especially do not want to give out one of the gems of Chinese civilization.

Though the vast majority of Chinese martial arts masters would not teach me the real stuff or would teach me incorrectly, the Taoists were beyond cultural and personal differences. They found it admirable that a Westerner would take the time and trouble to learn their language to be able to study something (Chi Gung) that they considered very important. The Taoists are generally highly developed spiritually, and considered the development of spiritual life to transcend time, space, and culture. The majority of in-depth Chi Gung work I have learned was taught to me by this group, and without them it would have been impossible for me to make sense of this subject.

Comparing Chi Gung Systems

One thing I saw very clearly during the course of my studies was that many types of Chi Gung consistently caused problems in a certain percentage of practitioners, while other types didn't seem to do all that much either positively or negatively. I also saw that some systems had broad applications, so that the same technique could be used to benefit many different problems, while some were very specific. Some systems mixed well with others, whereas some did not.

The following cases illustrate some of the difficulties that can arise from the improper practice of Chi Gung. In each of these cases I have either known the individual personally or the problem has actually occurred to me. I was extremely lucky that my first teacher, Wang Shu-Jin taught me only safe practices, but later on I learned a number of dangerous practices, some of which caused me great harm. Though I originally did not believe that Chi Gung could cause problems, I found out the hard way that it can.

Case 1: Too Much Chi Is Painful

My teacher Liu Hung Chieh passed on his Hsing I and Ba Gua lineage to one other person, Bai Hwa. Bai Hwa at one time taught in Amoy (Xiamen, Fukien Province), and this case concerns one of his students.

Bai Hwa taught this student the basic Hsing I Nei Gung practice of sinking the chi to the lower *tantien* (called the *hara* in Japanese and located in the lower abdomen) and after about two years of practice his student began to get very powerful. At this time Bai Hwa left Amoy for another city, and his student began to visit a number of Hsing I masters, looking for secret techniques from each. What he learned he practiced diligently, knowing that his first technique had worked so well.

Unfortunately his perseverance backfired. After a year practicing these techniques, though none were inherently bad, the combination resulted in all sorts of problems. In his effort to build chi in his lower *tantien* he ended up forcing his chi below his *tantien* and into his genitals. He effectively emptied the chi from his middle burner (internal organs) into his lower burner. This breaking of the natural energetic seal between the middle and lower burners left his middle burner chi in total disarray. This resulted in mental and physical problems, including involuntary semen emissions and hallucinations. He lost his job, and his impending marriage had to be postponed indefinitely.

It took an herbal master and Bai Hwa three years to bring him back to near normal. It takes much less time to do damage to your chi than to fix it. Imagine if this happened in America—the chance of finding genuine experts capable of treating his problems would be slim indeed.

Case 2: Sexual Chi Gung Can Be Dangerous

Many people today are fascinated by Chi Gung techniques for developing sexual power.

There is a system, for instance, that includes techniques such as forcibly sucking energy up the anus and spine and hanging weights of ever-increasing amounts from the testicles and penis.

My teacher Hung I Hsiang advised me fifteen years ago, when I mentioned this technique to him, that it would be a very bad idea for me to practice it. Wang Shu Jin, my first teacher and a man known for his Taoist sexual abilities, also warned me against it around 1970. In fact, I was given a one hour lecture from Hung I Hsiang on stupid chi practices, in which he cautioned about practicing esoteric sexual Chi Gung.

Lesser problems are even more common. I've met many people who practice sexual control techniques and damage their sexual apparatus. It is easy to overstrain the system, especially if the sexual organs are genetically weak to begin with. Some common problems include epididimitis (swollen testicles) and internal bleeding. While these practices may lead to the ability to maintain erections for a longer time, the increased pressure can damage the underlying tissues. Women, too, can be damaged by inappropriate sexual Chi Gung practices, resulting in problems such as false pregnancies and erratic periods.

For men, another sexual martial arts and Chi Gung practice that can cause problems involves sucking the testicles up into the body. Wang Shu-Jin advised me not to practice this technique because I was traveling too often, and he couldn't monitor me closely enough. He also said that, even with close monitoring a certain percentage of people are damaged by it, if the practice is begun after puberty.

Close supervision by a master is highly recommended when learning any sexual Chi Gung practices. America is now a workshop culture, where material that was traditionally presented over months is presented in a day or two or even an hour.

In Taoism, it is traditional to not teach dangerous material without all possible precautions. In some traditions, it is felt that if the majority is helped and only a minority may be harmed, overall more good than harm is being done. Anyone should be aware that they could be one of this minority, and you may not know until it is too late.

I will only publicly teach Chi Gung techniques that are virtually risk free. Only privately, where I can provide proper supervision, will I teach riskier material that has potentially faster results than the very safe techniques. In a way, the difference is like putting your money in a money market account, where growth is slow, steady, and sure, or playing fast and loose with your money in the stock market or commodities.

Case 3: The Downside of Packing Chi

Hung I Hsiang's brother was a practitioner of White Crane Chi Gung. A common technique of Shaolin Chi Gung methods such as White Crane is to force, or "pack," energy into the body, much like forcing clothes into a suitcase. This involves forceful breathing, body contractions, and a sense of physical and energetic strength. By overdoing it, Hung I Hsiang's brother actually caused one of his lungs to hemorrhage, and died.

In the West, I have seen people practicing all sorts of chi packing exercises, and these techniques are all potentially dangerous if not carefully supervised over time. Forceful packing can potentially cause damage to lung tissue, internal hemor-rhaging, imbalances in the overall body energy, and susceptibility to respiratory diseases.

A karate practitioner in her late forties came to see me in Boston, who because of practicing a packing exercise she had learned in a workshop, had had pneumonia for the last four winters. The practice she had learned was quite forceful. She had been perfectly healthy before. I found that she had been practicing incorrectly, but diligently. After I worked with her, she went through the next winter without getting pneumonia. Fortunately, her case was correctable, but many are not.

Another person, an assistant instructor of a well-known East Coast martial arts master, was told to practice the Small Heavenly (Microcosmic) Orbit in a forceful way, using reverse breathing to generate heat in the lower *tantien*, which was then circulated. This person was also told to squeeze his anus and forcibly lift his energy up his spine with his breathing.

The more he did this, the stronger and more powerful his energy felt. As in other Chi Gung techniques, the greater the force used, the stronger the experience generated. Unfortunately, he was burning himself up, especially his kidney and heart energy. When he began to experience symptoms such as cold, clammy sweats, involuntary tremors, extreme sensitivity to cold, and loss of vitality he was told to keep practicing, to "burn through the blockage." Even though he stopped these practices, it took more than five years of working on the problem to get rid of the symptoms.

The fact that these symptoms arose is not in itself dire, since they could have been corrected at an early stage. His teacher failed to pay attention to the warning signals and, instead, made the student feel that there was something wrong with him! If your body or mind experiences great difficulties when you practice Chi Gung, simply stop. The trouble may not reside in you, but rather in faulty teaching or your misunderstanding the instructions.

Case 4: Vibrating Chi (Crane Styles)

In many Chi Gung systems, especially Shaolin-style and animal styles (White Crane, for example) there is a technique that deliberately tries to vibrate chi in the body. The breath oscillates rapidly, and chi is vibrated inside bones, tissues, brain, and so forth.

This type of practice may have a number of unpleasant side effects. It can make a person absolutely uncaring, and, as the vibrations get stronger, it can bring on a kind of megalomania, or other mental illnesses. It can also cause physical hallucinations, where sensations of shaking, opening, and closing continue after practice has stopped. And if these practices are continued long enough, they can cause problems in the internal organs. The lungs and liver are the most vulnerable, but the other organs are susceptible as well.

It is quite common in these practices for the chi to be incompletely or irregularly circulated, rather than fully awakened and circulated. When I first saw these vibrating practices in Beijing, it was very obvious that the way they were forcing chi was causing what in India would be called irregularly awakened kundalini.

My medical Chi Gung teacher in Beijing informed me that these types of vibratory practices historically had a high casualty rate. She had worked with cancer patients who had brought their symptoms under control with Chi Gung and then begun vibratory practices, which brought their cancer out of remission, and they returned to the hospital to die. The strong sense of power makes these practices addictive, and like crack, when the crash comes, it is too late.

When I was 21 I was taught a "secret" technique. I was told it was the Chi Gung that was the power behind Tai Chi. I practiced this technique diligently, two hours a day, until I was able to break bones with one slap simply by vibrating my energy. At the same time, I noticed an incredibly seductive feeling of energy in my head, and I began to realize that I was becoming psychotic. The stronger this chi got, the stranger my mind became, and the hotter my body felt.

In a particularly raucous martial art incident in Japan, I found I was breaking bones left and right, and was almost unable to stop myself. At this point, I realized this practice was making me crazy, removing compassion from my makeup, and I stopped. When I later returned to Taiwan a few years later, I found I had been practicing the Tsung He form of Fukien White Crane, and that some of the practitioners of this art were either subtly or obviously psychotic. Many of the most humble-seeming masters of this Chi Gung were actually the most dangerous. Power replaced compassion, and while they might use their power for healing, it would be of little concern to them if they accidentally caused damage instead.

A student of Tai Chi in San Diego (let's call him Mike) studied with an instructor who taught a form that involved vibrating the mind, body, and breath. He was in his teens at the time, with no martial arts background, and thought this was traditional Tai Chi Chuan. His first year felt good and relaxed, but then his teacher wanted to increase his pace. Weapon forms and more breathing practices were added to increase the vibration. About two-and-a-half years into his training, he developed the ability to discharge energy on a crude level, and he felt he was really coming along. Unfortunately, he also began to notice some side effects. These included (1) frightening hallucinations of his consciousness leaving his body and drifting uncontrollably away; (2) feeling that things were moving much faster than they actually were (this was especially dangerous when he was driving); (3) feeling his body become stiffer and stiffer internally; (4) developing a thirst for power; (5) feeling constantly hyper, unable to calm down; and (6) experiencing involuntary body spasms.

These problems were also beginning to happen to a friend of his, who happened to come to one of my classes. I noticed that he was essentially shredding himself, and taught him to drain and repattern this vibrational energy. He in turn told his friend to come and see me.

By this time Mike had not been practicing for three years, yet most of his symptoms had not abated. He literally feared for his mental and physical health. I found that he had condensed the chi in his body, and through various techniques I repatterned his energy and taught him how to continue this process at home. I also taught him techniques for removing the damaging chi from his body, techniques very similar to those found in this book. Two years later, his problems had pretty much dissolved.

Discharging Energy

Many other Chi Gung practices, such as discharging energy at a distance, are not inherently dangerous but do require a firm foundation in the grounding techniques described in this book. Most problems in Chi Gung are the result of energy getting stuck, energy not flowing through the system, Knowing how to ground energy out can be a lifesaver. I should also add that much of the time, the action-at-a-distance Chi Gung requires a good deal of cooperation among the participants, and there is a certain amount of exaggeration going on whenever this subject is discussed or demonstrated. These are methods for training a person's sensitivity to chi. It is virtually impossible to make a person with a developed will to move or jump against his or her will by only projecting chi at a distance without physical contact.

The Dangers of Forcing and Fast Results

Chi Gung practices that give you a very rapid sense of increased physical or psychic power sometimes do so by overstraining the central nervous system. Chi Gung systems that promote an even, steady, upward curve of chi development are safer and usually more reliable for longterm progress. Extreme, forceful practices have the most consistently dangerous side-effects. If you undertake forceful practices, you should be supervised—by regular ongoing weekly contact with a teacher who can adjust chi development to turn a potentially dangerous practice into a safe one. Many Shaolin practices are extremely forceful, so a good, ethical, honest, experienced and knowledgeable teacher is a necessity.

If your body, mind, emotions, or psychic perceptions are getting weird or painful simply *stop practicing* until you find out clearly what is going on. Whatever your strength or capacity, your Chi Gung practices must be internally comfortable. Forcing yourself radically beyond your individual limitations is usually what causes damage to your nerves, glands, internal organs, and brain. Overdoing internal energy practices may be compared to the overtraining that causes external body damage in athletes. First and foremost find an experienced, ethical, competent teacher who has your best interests at heart.

Most Chi Gung Is Safe

Notwithstanding all the previous warnings, most Chi Gung systems are actually quite safe. Don't be afraid to practice Chi Gung simply because some techniques may be dangerous. All valuable technologies have some element of danger. The purpose of this Appendix is simply to open people's eyes to the negative aspects of Chi Gung, which are commonly glossed over in our infatuation with things strange and foreign. I wish to reiterate that the material presented in this book and other volumes in the series is the safest and most effective I have found in over twenty years of research.

Appendix D
Origin of Material
in This Book

In 1968, I learned the outer form—the physical shell—of most material taught in this volume from my teacher Wang Shu-Jin in Taiwan and his student Chang I Jung in Tokyo. I practiced this material five hours a day for five months, and then over the next eighteen years learned the internal components from various teachers and Taoist masters, including Hung I Hsiang and Huang Hsi I.

The standing posture is the most basic posture in Chi Gung, and is found to some degree in all schools. It is the Taoist equivalent to the martial arts horse stance.

Cloud Hands is the basic exercise to connect the arms and legs to the spine. The First Swing, which energizes the lower organs, is found in almost all Chi Gung systems. The Second Swing, which joins the legs to the spine and energizes the middle organs, is less common, and the Third Swing, which energizes the upper organs and the brain, is less common still. Historically, though, they were done together and, from an energetic perspective, they should be done together. One swing alone may not be strong enough to cure a serious problem, but when done together and in the order presented, the effect is synergistic.

The spinal stretch was the only movement I did not originally learn from Wang, but it has been traditionally (for 3000 years) included in this sequence. It is the beginning move of traditional spinal Chi Gung. In its entirety, spinal Chi Gung teaches how to bring energy up the spine, connect the spine to the rest of the body, completely control vertebral movement, and access the cerebro-spinal pump, which purely deals with the spine.

About one-half of the internal components of these exercises have been included in this volume, and the rest of the internal matrix can be found in forthcoming volumes of this series, including the Spiraling Energy Body. Some of the internal energetic work, it should be pointed out, can only safely be learned under the supervision of a master,* and I have only included here what can be presented to the general public without danger.

I had the help of many masters, some of whom I cannot mention by name because of the political situation in China. Others I cannot mention because it was their expressed wish to depart the world "without leaving any footprints." I could, however, never have gotten the complete picture without having been formally adopted by Liu Hung Chieh and accepted as his disciple. Liu filled in the gaps in my education, as well as teaching me much less common material; material that came from his ten years learning with Taoist adepts in the mountains of Western China, rather than from his martial arts background.

Liu Hung Chieh's Education as a Taoist Master

Liu Hung Chieh began to study martial arts at the age of 12. After three years of training in Shaolin-style Kung Fu, he was accepted as the youngest formal disciple by the Beijing Ba Gua school. At this time, he also learned Hsing I from members of the school and outside teachers. In 1928, he represented the Beijing Ba Gua school at the first All China Martial Arts Competition, which had to be stopped due to excessive injuries.

In the mid-1930s, Liu was head of instructors at the Hunan Branch of the Central Government's National Martial Arts Association. Two of his junior instructors at that time were Wu Jien Chuan's sons, and from them he learned Wu style Tai Chi. Later, Liu became Wu Jien Chuan's formal disciple, and lived in Wu's house in Hong Kong. Because of Liu's strong internal martial arts background, Wu was able to teach him the deepest levels of the Wu style.

When Liu returned to the mainland he studied with the abbot Tan Hsu Fa Shi, and was declared formally enlightened ac-

Editor's Note: Due to the depth of the material in the Spiraling Energy Body, Kumar Frantzis teaches it only during annual week-long summer retreats.

cording to the tenets of Tien Tai Buddhism. He then spent ten years studying with Taoist masters in Szechuan Province in Western China, completing the practice for becoming one with the Tao.

With the ascension of Communism in China, he returned to Beijing, where he lived out the rest of his life quietly, teaching only a few students, and perfecting his practices.

Appendix E
About the Romanization of Chinese Words in This Book

Any attempt to transliterate the sounds of Chinese words into English with any accuracy will fall far short. This is because Chinese not only has sounds that English does not have, but it uses a system of vocal "tones," which do not exist in English. Furthermore, English has sounds that are not present in Chinese. English speakers attempting to pronounce Chinese words will invariably add sounds from their own language, which will distort the pronunciation of Chinese.

None of the major systems for Romanizing Chinese words is very accurate. Written Chinese is composed of ideogram pictures, each of which may convey one idea or several combined ideas. These ideograms, when spoken, are pronounced differently in the different Chinese languages. To the foreign ear, these languages can sometimes seem as different as French and German. For example, the word for family is *jia* in the "National Language" (Mandarin, or common-people speech), but it is *gar* in Cantonese (a regional Chinese sublanguage, or dialect, spoken by over sixty million people in the province of Canton and by the people of Hong Kong). There are yet more regional languages, again with different sounds for the same character, such as Szechuanese (which more people speak than Cantonese) and Minnanhua of Fukien province (which is an older language than

Cantonese). To make matters worse, there are subdialects within each major dialect. In some instances in Old China, people from the same province only one or two hundred miles away from each other could hardly communicate with each other. (Bear in mind that China is a very big place.)

This linguistic mess stymied communication throughout China for thousands of years, with the written language (in a mostly illiterate nation) being the only common means of communication. As all power in Old China came from the Emperor and his bureaucracy, over time the language of Beijing became the common medium of communication throughout China for the educated. After the Emperors fell, both the Nationalist government and, later, the Communist government made the language of Beijing—still the seat of government—the national language of China and called it the Common People's speech, which, in English, is called Mandarin Chinese (from the days of the Emperors). Mandarin, as the official language of all of China, is now what truly can be called Chinese, which every single person in China learns to speak. Throughout this book, all Chinese terms used are in Mandarin and not in the regional dialects.

The Westerner who has no idea how to speak Chinese (and probably little interest in learning) is now bombarded with multiple systems of transliteration for the exact same sound, including the Pin Yin system, the Wade-Giles system, and the Yale system. In both the Wade-Giles system (invented by German monks, used in the old days by translators who mostly could only read Chinese but not speak it, and now used by the Nationalists in Taiwan), and the Pin Yin system (developed for use inside China by the Chinese when the Communist government was trying to raise the literacy rate in China), many of the written English words when pronounced do not sound anything like the Chinese sounds. The only Romanization system that was created to mimic as closely as possible the Chinese language using the English phonetic system was the Yale system, created at Yale University specifically to teach English speakers how to speak Chinese.

For example, *Chi Gung* in the Yale system is *Chi Gung*; in Pin Yin, it is *Qi Gong*; and in Wade-Giles, it is *Chi Kung*. Actually, the way it is said in China is closest to *Chee Gung*. The *Qi* of the Pin Yin and the *Kung* of the Wade-Giles are not accurate.

This language lesson may seem academic to some. However, there are over a billion Chinese in the world and miscommunication can waste a lot of time and energy. This book uses transliterations that allow the English speaker to best mimic what the Chinese actually sounds like. Thus, I have not been concerned with adhering strictly to any one formal transliteration system.

Appendix F
The Taoist Energy System Taught by Bruce Kumar Frantzis

Taoist Energy Enhancement Practices for Health, Healing, Self-Defense, and Spiritual Advancement

Do you want to have more energy in your life to improve your health, to heal others, to protect yourself against physical violence, or to advance your spirituality? Bruce Kumar Frantzis spent ten years in China thoroughly learning the Taoist way of using the energy of the body for these purposes.

Mr. Frantzis now offers a complete system of Taoist practices for achieving these goals. This system of Taoist internal work demystifies these esoteric practices and gives you direct access to them.

Master the Energy of the Body—Core Practices

Six basic Chi Gung (energy enhancement) courses teach the fundamental processes of moving energy within the body. Those who develop a full understanding of these basics will much more easily achieve their potential in the more advanced work and applications. (Mr. Frantzis is currently writing a book for each of these courses.)

- **Dragon and Tiger Chi Gung and Standing Meditation** Easy to learn. Quickly gives you a recognizable feeling of energy in your body. Invigorating and calming. Release stress and pain. Recommended for beginners.
- **Opening the Energy Gates of Your Body** Establishes the physical alignments necessary for maximum energy flow and efficient movement. Can prevent injuries during any type of exercise.
- **The Joining of Heaven and Earth** Circulates energy through the entire body. Strengthens, heals and increases the elasticity of your joints. Reveals the secrets of Taoist breathing. Enables you to project energy from your hands for healing yourself or others.
- **Bend the Bow and Shoot the Arrow** Puts a spring in your spine that most people have not experienced since they were teenagers. Heals chronic back problems. Improves posture. Overhauls and strengthens your central nervous system.
- **Spiraling Energy Body** Can raise your energy level dramatically. Teaches you to master how energy moves in circles and spirals through your body. Enables you to project energy to any part of your body at will.
- **Gods Playing in the Clouds** Combines all of the benefits of the above exercises. Cleanses and stabilizes the central channel of energy in the body. Makes the bones harder and stronger. Energizes the brain. Clears negative emotions from the body.

Improve Your Physical and Emotional Health

To repair injuries, strengthen your body, decrease stress, and increase resistance to disease, you should study the following courses, in addition to the six Core Practices. These advanced movement arts intensify the benefits of the six Core Practices.

- **Wu Style Tai Chi Short Form** This Tai Chi form develops flexibility, coordination, gracefulness, ease of movement and stamina. Particularly beneficial for healing injuries, especially back problems. Consists of a sequence of eighteen choreographed movements, practiced in a slow meditative manner.

- **Ba Gua Single Palm Change** A vigorous and aerobic, yet relaxed, practice based on walking in a circle, and frequently changing direction. Makes your body extremely strong, flexible and graceful, and enables you to move with lightning speed and unpredictability. Gives you vibrant health.

Heal Others

The six Core Practices or equivalent Chi Gung experiences are prerequisites for:

- **Chi Gung Tui Na** Project energy from your hands, voice and eyes into other people to unblock and balance their energy and facilitate healing. You can combine this energy work with any of hundreds of Chinese bodywork/massage techniques, including deep tissue, joint and lymph work, acupressure, nerve release work, and internal organ realignment.
- **Chi Gung Therapy** Use specific standing postures and Chi Gung exercises to alter energy flows or blockages contributing to particular physical, emotional, and mental health problems.

Protect Yourself Against Physical Violence

Instruction is offered in the following martial arts:

- **Tai Chi Chuan** When practicing Tai Chi as a martial art, you move at blinding speed using circular movements which turn the energy of opponents back on them. B. K. Frantzis teaches the complete traditional systems of both the Wu and Yang Styles of Tai Chi Chuan, including long forms, push hands, self defense techniques and weapons.
- **Hsing I Chuan** Use internal energy to deliver powerful linear punches and blocks, while aggressively stealing your opponents' strength or overwhelming them.
- **Ba Gua Chang** Specializes in circular footwork and spiraling, constant movement. Disappear like a ghost from your opponents' strikes and unpredictably deliver blows from any direction at any time. Fight eight opponents simultaneously. Ba Gua also is a Taoist moving meditation art.

Learn to Evolve Spiritually Toward the Tao

Lao Tse's Traditional Water Meditation Method was taught to B. K. Frantzis in Beijing by the late Taoist sage Liu Hung Chieh. (Lao Tse wrote the *Tao Te Ching*.) The philosophical basis of most Eastern energy-based meditation methods introduced to the West is that of the Yang way of fire, in which you reach spiritual and physical advancement by forcing through obstacles. Conversely, in Lao Tse's Yin way of water, spiritual obstacles are dissolved.

The I Ching Method of Meditation is an essential part of the Yin way of water. You learn to experience and bring into your body and mind the eight essential energies of the universe, which are described by the eight trigrams of the *I Ching: The Book of Changes*.

Taoist Internal Alchemy Practices enable you to transform the energy of your body into the essential energies of the universe. You learn to use all the body's energy channels and centers, especially the three Tantien centers or elixir fields.

B. K. Frantzis teaches practices to help you through two of the three stages of this Taoist approach to spiritual realization.

Attain Stillness: The Preliminary Practices

Work toward Jing (stillness), in which the energies of the body and emotions become stable. Achieve a quiet mind, greater capacity for patience and perseverance, freedom from obsessions, good health, and the ability to handle stress by learning the following practices.

- **Transmute Your Physical Body**   Dissolve the physical and emotional energy blockages of the body, and transform the internal organs and glands to a superior level of function.
- **Gain Emotional Maturity**   Clear yourself of those energies and conditionings in your body and mind that bind you. Enjoy sexual meditation practices that open your energy channels and bring internal harmony to your relationships.
- **Invoke the Energies of Heaven and Earth**   Taoist "shamanistic" practices tap into the energies of heaven and earth, and the five elements of metal, water, wood, earth, and fire. Obtain these from the environment—trees, oceans, people,

mountains, planets, and stars—and use them as sources for your transformational work.

- **Integrate Stillness with Movement**   Integrate these internal meditation practices into movement arts, such as Tai Chi and Ba Gua.

Spiritual Rebirth: The Mature Practices

Taoist alchemy focuses on the middle and upper energy centers of your body; the heart and brain.

- **Open Your Heart**   Open your heart to its higher potentials of universal balance, equanimity, kindness, love, and compassion.
- **Open Your Mind**   By opening your mind, you can learn to discriminate between the real and the false, understand the energies that cause events, and gain admittance to the unseen world of the cosmos.
- **Open Your Soul**   Raise and merge the energies of your body, heart, and mind to become one with yourself, awakening your true spiritual nature and entering a world beyond words.

The Tao

As a newly born spiritual being, evolve on the journey of becoming one with all the universe. Unlike the previous two stages, this one does not require specific practices. Each individual's way become Self-apparent. Each spiritual being ultimately matures and becomes one with the Tao as an immortal sage.

How You Can Learn More

While this book is an excellent introduction to Chi Gung, it is not a substitute for personal instruction. B. K. Frantzis offers you many ways to explore his system of Taoist Energy Enhancement Practices for health, healing, self-defense, and spiritual advancement.

- **Summer Retreats**   The ideal way to learn is to go on a one- to two-week retreat in a beautiful California location. Study with B. K. Frantzis and make friends with other students in a serene atmosphere conducive to learning and relaxation: a wonderful vacation, as well! (Winter retreats may also be offered.)
- **Weekend Workshops**   For a first-time experience or for on-going study, Mr. Frantzis teaches workshops regularly in the San Francisco area, New York, Boston, and London. He and senior instructors also are available to teach in other cities in the United States and Europe.
- **Instructor Trainings**   For those interested in becoming certi-fied instructors, these classes are held in the San Francisco area and can last from ten days to two months. A senior instructor training institute is being established, with courses of study that last one to three years.
- **Ongoing Classes**   B. K. Frantzis and his instructors teach weekly classes in the San Francisco area. There are other on-going classes in Massachusetts, New York, Florida, New Mexico, and Arizona, as well as in Great Britain.
- **Videotapes**   Subjects range from B. K. Frantzis's general in-troduction to Taoist practices, to specific topics such as Open-ing the Energy Gates and Tai Chi Self-Defense Techniques. (Volume discounts available.)

For more information, please send the enclosed postcard to B.K. Frantzis, P.O. Box 99, Fairfax, California 94978-0099, USA. ☎ (415) 454–5243

Photo and Art Credits

Photos

Front Cover © 1993 David Hiser/The Image Bank.

Back Cover Anthony Ortega.

Page ii Ken Van Sickle.

Acknowledgments *Page x:* Caroline Frantzis.

Foreword *Page xvi:* Caroline Frantzis.
Page xxii: Ken Van Sickle. *Page xxvi:* Sara Barchus.

Chapter 2 *Page 24:* Caroline Frantzis.

Chapter 3 *Page 44:* Caroline Frantzis.

Chapter 6 *Page 94:* Anthony Ortega.

Chapter 9 *Page 120:* Hideki Matsuoka.

Art

Cover Design: Paula Goldstein, Bookman Productions.

Interior Design: Suzanne Montazer, Bookman Productions.

Illustrations: Kurt Schulten, Husky Grafx.

B. K. Frantzis Energy Arts
Mastery without Mystery™

B. K. Frantzis Energy Arts offers corporate programs, instructor trainings, weekend seminars and week-long retreats in the United States and Europe. Books, audiotapes and videotapes to support these teachings are available through:

B. K. Frantzis Energy Arts®
P. O. Box 99
Fairfax, California 94978-0099
USA
Phone: (415) 454-5243
Fax: (415) 454-0907
Website: www.energyarts.com

Other books by B. K. Frantzis:

The Power of Internal Martial Arts: Combat Secrets of Ba Gua, Tai Chi and Hsing-I (North Atlantic Books, Berkeley, CA) 1998. Available in bookstores.

The Water Method of Taoist Meditation Series:
Vol. I: *Relaxing into Your Being*, (Clarity Press, Fairfax, CA) 1998.
Vol. II: *The Great Stillness* (Clarity Press, Fairfax, CA) 1999.
Available through B. K. Frantzis Energy Arts.

For more information, tear out and mail the postcard on the next page.